Life on th Reflux Roller Coaster

Gastro Esophageal Reflux Disease in Infants and Children

Written by
Roni MacLean
and
Jean McNeil

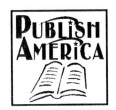

PublishAmerica
Baltimore

First printing

ISBN: 1-4137-0833-1
PUBLISHED BY PUBLISHAMERICA, LLLP
www.publishamerica.com
Baltimore

Printed in the United States of America

Dedicated to:

Shae-Lynne
My gift from God.
Thank you for all you have taught me and all you have given me. You are truly the greatest joy in my life. I am proud of you and I love you to the moon and back.

And to the thousands of infants who know the pains of
GERD
May a cure be soon found.

In Loving Memory

Eric Charles Hayes
April 5, 1973 - Mar 24, 2002

Alicia Toms
May 15, 1977 - Dec 1, 1991

Robert Peter Hayes, Jr.
Feb 1, 1972 - Jan 30, 1988

They left us too soon.

Comments about *Life on the Reflux Roller Coaster*

This is a story of a frustrated family dealing with an adorable daughter failing to grow properly due to GERD. Her mother's frustration with the diagnosis, treatment, and medical system responsible for caring for her daughter is evident. Its intent is to assure other families with children in similar situations that they are not alone. While it is important families in situations like these research the diseases, keep in mind you should always consult your physician before trying any suggestion that concerns your child's health. Use your research to be able to ask appropriate questions, and seek second opinions without fear of offending the doctor—any doctor comfortable with his/her ability should welcome a second opinion. But keep your options open, and while stories like these are wonderful for emotional support, they do not serve as a basis to make medical decisions—everyone is different. That being said, the emotional support this lends may be the critical factor in coping with your child's illness, and should not be underestimated.

David Earle, M.D.
Director of Minimally Invasive Surgery
Bay State Medical Center
Springfield, MA, USA
Assistant Professor of Surgery
Tufts University School of Medicine

Disclaimer:

I am not a medical professional, just a mother. I hold no degrees in medicine. The information provided in this book comes from my own research into this disease. I provide this information only to help you to be as informed as possible when dealing with medical professionals. Do not try anything suggested in this book without first consulting your child's doctor.

Roni MacLean

ACKNOWLEDGMENTS

Thanks to Duncan…who, although he probably doesn't remember, told me I could write.

Thanks to Jim MacDonald for his encouraging support at the beginning, helping us to believe in the reality of our book.

Thanks to Karen, Nikki, Katey, and Christy for reading. Their constructive criticism and positive feedback were very welcomed.

Thank you to both William Greenleaf and Florence Stearns for donating your time by reading and editing one of our many drafts. May Mrs. Stearns forever be blessed with this gift.

Thanks to Dr. David Earle, Dr. Bernie Siegel and Rick Bell. We sincerely appreciate the time you took from your busy schedules to read and contribute to our story.

Dr. Doris Rapp took the time from writing her own book *Our Toxic World— A Wake Up Call* to read our draft. She is an incredibly awesome lady and we are truly grateful for her taking part in our book.

A special thank you to Shae-Lynne's doctors. Throughout this book it may sound as though I didn't like Shae's team of doctors and much frustration with their lack of help is expressed. Now I know they have done everything medically possible. After reading other parents' stories about how their reflux kids are treated (or not treated) and how little there pediatricians seem to know about reflux, I am all the more grateful to Shae-Lynne's doctor. I believe that we got lucky to have such wonderful doctors and she has gotten the best care possible for a child with her condition. My frustration now lies where it belongs, in the disease and the lack of options for treatment.

We realize how extremely difficult it may have been to share their personal story; to that extent we give praise and thanks to Greta, Claudia, Melissa, Lucy, Julie, Sonia and Patti.

Thanks to all the online reflux moms who helped me survive in the beginning and shared so much of their wisdom and support. Many of these women have more than one sick child and they have been doing this for years and years with no end in site. Their strength astounds me. To Lori and Susan I am particularly grateful. I think of all my friends on the message boards often and will never forget any of them, despite the fact that I seldom have time to visit them anymore. Ladies, here's praying for a day when there is no need for reflux support groups.

LIFE ON THE
REFLUX ROLLER COASTER

*Gastro Esophageal Reflux Disease
in Infants and Children*

TABLE OF CONTENTS

FOREWORD

This book is written for all the mothers who have been there. It is not only for the mothers of infants and children diagnosed with esophageal reflux. This illness is also present in a growing number of adults.[1] It is for all those parents who are desperate because they have a baby who is in pain and not normal. They cannot stand to see their lovely child suffer another minute, yet it goes on and on. They see light at the end of the tunnel but it repeatedly goes out and the pain and suffering barely leaves before it is back. They are afraid to complain because they fear they will receive no further help and they do not know where to turn. They are asked to wait for test results, for appointments, for explanations when there are really no good reasons. They are shunted from doctor to doctor, each saying the other will resolve the problem—or even worse, saying nothing. They are asked to make decisions when they have little understanding of the pros and cons and they do not know whom to ask or where to go for an impartial opinion.

They only know their child is suffering now and they need to know if their baby will suffer even more after the next treatment, medication or procedure that is supposed to help. The never-ending disappointments leave them feeling inadequate, helpless, angry, fearful and exhausted. The following expresses how I personally felt after reading this most informative and candid "how to" book that is a must for every parent of a reflux infant or child.

I believe the author's main purpose for this book is to express that there isn't a cure. Gastro esophageal reflux in infants, as well as adults, is a disease—just like diabetes or any other chronic disease. Because reflux is so common and widespread, it is difficult to believe that something so benign and usually easily treatable could wreak such havoc, make someone seriously ill and in some cases not be treatable or curable. Therefore, each reader must realize that this is a potentially serious disease for which, at present time, there are certainly no easy answers or cures—but some improvement is indeed possible.

What is the answer for parents of infants with reflux?[2a, b] First, totally forget the guilt. You have in all probability gone far above and beyond in every way that is humanly possible as the mother of Shae-Lynne so vividly describes in this book. The last thing you should do is blame yourself. You have a right to be upset and to express it. You have a right to be tired and exhausted when you are unwell or have not been able to sleep or eat properly for short or prolonged periods of time because you are caring for your sick child and neglecting yourself and your needs. You have a right to be too tired to care properly for all the other facets of your life that you know also need love and attention. You have a right to be concerned about the endless bills you cannot pay and the progressively depleted funds. You have a right to be concerned about vomiting, choking, turning blue, tubes, sore skin areas, dressings and endless screaming in pain that is not remotely similar to crying. You have a very sick child!

Secondly, you need to know that unfortunately you are not alone. Many others have gone through exactly the same anguish, wondering and worrying about their sick, precious, helpless, suffering, darling child. Mothers and fathers of children with GERD have been there and done that. They know. They have seen the many specialists, tried the many medications, had the multiple surgeries to correct the original problem, plus the new ones created by the latest or previous surgeries. They must be aware that surgically treated infants will have great difficulty learning to swallow or chew normally after the Nissen fundoplication procedure is performed. It is not easy to accept, but parents must know that the opening in the stomach will eventually have to be stretched and the surgery may have to be revised. Mothers such as Shae-Lynne's have not only exhausted themselves, but also their spouses, their families and their finances. They and their child need compassion, understanding, and most of all, explanations and help. This book provides some insight as to what can and does happen in the real world of reflux therapy. It can increase the awareness of parents who are also at a crossroads trying to decide which direction to follow.

Thirdly, this book made me ask, what can a physician do to help? The key question is why is this happening?[1, 2c] Nothing is simple in medicine and there are certainly many possible causes for children who are not normal at birth and who have a medical problem such as GERD. It helps if you can find a doctor who you know has treated infants with the type of medical problems your child has.[3] Find one who will take the time to explain what has happened to your child and will patiently and compassionately detail what might be helpful and why. This is not easy but it can be done. Don't hesitate to switch doctors if you find you have the wrong one.

Doctors tend to see the part of the elephant they know most about. I am no exception.[2a-c] As I read this book the medical facts fell easily into my part of the elephant. The damaging pollution of our world could be one cause of reflux infants.[2c] This illness could easily have started when the babies were in the uterus filled with fluid that contained toxic chemicals.[2] How often has anyone checked these infants for toxic chemicals or metals? This exposure could have damaged their immune system, making them prone to allergies, especially to foods and recurrent infections.[2c] After birth, their feeding problems are exceptionally bad, so they are put on a hypo-allergenic formula.[2a] They develop a sensitivity or allergy to their first formula, or this occurs shortly after it is started. They are given another and it does not take long before this too is not tolerated. The same thing happens with the next formula that is tried. The milk, soy or corn (dextrose) eventually can all become a problem.

This statement is not written in cement but, in general, any food or formula that is repeatedly fed to an allergic infant or child will tend to similarly cause allergies in time. If your child fits into this category the answer is to rotate types of formulas and foods at least at a four-day interval.[4] Try allergy injection therapy for foods from environmental medical specialists.[2b] Most allergists do not believe it is possible but this type of treatment can definitely help some to many of the children who have this type of problem.

You might ask: Which GERD infants might have allergies as a major factor in relation to their illness? The answer: Those who have allergies in themselves or their other children.

Now for a second statement not written in cement. If infants are fed a formula or food *to which there is sensitivity*, they will vomit through the mouth. If the tube is put in the stomach, they will vomit through the stomach. If the tube is placed in the small intestine, they will vomit through that tube, but with a bit less gusto because the intestines have weaker muscles than the stomach. In an allergic infant if you eliminate the offending food, the vomiting will stop. If an infant pushes away the breast or a milk or soy formula, but appears to want food, feed the baby the tolerated foods.[5] The infant has given you the answer. But, remember, if the same food is fed repeatedly, every day, a sensitivity will develop to that food and eventually also will cause vomiting. Again, food allergy extract therapy might be an answer.

In summary, the best solution to this problem is prevention. If chemical pollution is the reason this illness is becoming more common, it must be recognized and corrected. If formulas and foods are contributing to an infant's suffering at least find out if the child can be treated with an allergy extract. If so, this might be the best answer. If the immune system is weak, use nutrients to strengthen it. If the infant's body contains toxic chemicals or metals, help him/her to detoxify or get rid of these harmful substances. If digestive enzymes are needed, give them. If these measures are effective, they can provide short- and long-term answers for those specific babies. Pollution and allergies are not the reasons for all infants with reflux, but they certainly are for some. If your child is one of these infants it is possible that there is both hope and help for your infant—and you.

Doris J Rapp., M.D.
Board certified pediatrician, allergist, and environmental medical specialist.

References

1. *No More Heartburn*, Sherry Rogers, MD

2. Books by Dr. Doris Rapp
   Environmental Research Foundation 800-787-8780
   a. *Is This Your Child*
   b. *Is This Your Child's World—Or Yours?*
   c. *Our Toxic World—A Wake Up Call*

3. Sally Rockwell, PhD, Rotation Diet Info 206-547-1814

4. AAEM 316-684-5500

5. Audiotape on infant allergies 716-875-0398

WELCOME TO HOLLAND

I am often asked to describe the experience of raising a child with a disability—to try to help people who have not shared that unique experience to understand it, to imagine how it would feel. It's like this....

When you're going to have a baby, it's like planning a fabulous vacation trip—to Italy. You buy a bunch of guidebooks and make your wonderful plans. The Coliseum. The Michelangelo *David*. The gondolas in Venice. You may learn some handy phrases in Italian. It's all very exciting.

After months of eager anticipation, the day finally arrives. You pack your bags and off you go. Several hours later, the plane lands. The stewardess comes in and says, "Welcome to Holland."

"Holland?!" you say. "What do you mean Holland? I signed up for Italy! I'm supposed to be in Italy. All my life I've dreamed of going to Italy."

But there's been a change in the flight plan. They've landed in Holland and there you must stay.

The important thing is that they haven't taken you to a horrible, disgusting, filthy place, full of pestilence, famine and disease. It's just a different place.

So you must go out and buy new guidebooks. And you must learn a whole new language. And you will meet a whole new group of people you would never have met.

It's just a different place. It's slower paced than Italy, less flashy than Italy. But after you've been there for a while and you catch your breath, you look around...and you begin to notice that Holland has windmills...and Holland has tulips. Holland even has Rembrandts.

But everyone you know is busy coming and going from Italy...and they're all bragging about what a wonderful time they had there. And for the rest of your life, you will say, "Yes, that's where I was supposed to go. That's what I had planned."

And the pain of that will never, ever, ever, ever go away...because the loss of that dream is a very, very significant loss.

But...if you spend your life mourning the fact that you didn't get to Italy, you may never be free to enjoy the very special, the very lovely things...about Holland.

INTRODUCTION

How can I—driving my car to work/taking a shower/lying in bed—contemplate writing Shae-Lynne's story and at the same time nine hundred miles away my daughter, Roni, is forming the same idea in her mind?

We are one heart, one soul, and two minds that have joined together in thought to share this story. Our thoughts reach across the miles; we know this story must be told. We share our story/*your* story. We have been there and we are still there. Infant Gastro Esophageal Reflux Disease (GERD) must be taken seriously. In a book that I have read recently by Elaine Shimberg, *Coping with Chronic Heartburn*, Ms. Shimberg quotes NORD (National Organization for Rare Disease). They explain that infant reflux is on the rise and that in 1992 this disease in infants was considered rare; however, by 1996 it had become one of the most common medical problems in infants. Some infants do not outgrow this as quickly as expected and they continue to be affected until their second birthday or even into adolescence.

It is a very misunderstood and often difficult disease to diagnose. You may have heard of it as being referred to as heartburn in adults. Believe me, what we write about is a far cry from heartburn. We wish to bring awareness to what these infants and families are going through. An adult can express what he is feeling, where he hurts. When an infant is involved, we can only guess.

We were lucky and appreciated that Shae-Lynne's pediatrician, Dr. Andrews, was very sympathetic. He seemed to really care. He even called after hours just to see how Shae-Lynne was doing. In the beginning, he didn't seem to have any answers. We could feel his frustration. "This is a mystery to me," we heard several times.

From the day Shae-Lynne was born she would not eat. She gagged and retched, not as a normal baby that spits up. I mean she actually choked. Sometimes she stopped breathing; it was extremely difficult to watch. It was not until Shae-Lynne turned four months old (and after more trips to the hospital than I care to remember) that she was finally diagnosed with GERD. There were no books written on what we were experiencing. If there were any chapters on this subject the final note was "if the problem is severe call your doctor." Well, we were seeing the doctor almost daily for the increasingly stressful weigh in. Each day we were more disappointed as Shae-Lynne's weight was down more than up.

Life on the Reflux Roller Coaster was written so that you will not have to go through the long drawn-out process that we have. It is written so that you will gain knowledge from our struggle. In a concise, easy-to-read format this part of your journey in life will be made easier by following Shae-Lynne's story.

Yes, Gastro Esophageal Reflux Disease (GERD) is very serious. This book is about the horrors of watching your infant/child: (1) not eat, (2) vomit uncontrollably, (3) fail to thrive, and (4) cry out continually in pain while you just watch. It is about learning to cope, while others simply do not understand. It is about the frustration felt every time someone says, "Oh, it is only reflux, she will grow out of it." I wonder, *has their child been hospitalized most of their short life? Has their child just been cut open to have a feeding tube inserted? Have they held their drugged child in their arms after a three-hour operation?* No, I don't think I want to hear, "Oh, it is only reflux, she will grow out of it." I guess we are led to believe that if an infant is born with GERD eventually they will grow out of it. Hearing this does not help when you are living this hell and trying to get through each hour—that happens to be lasting into a year or more!

It is time *infant* GERD come out in the open. It's like infant GERD is being hid in the closet that no one sees, or will admit is there. Inside, unseen, it burns away at the esophagus causing considerable damage. Gastro Esophageal Reflux Disease is here and it is on the rise. It has increased dramatically in the last ten years.

Although I am not with Shae-Lynne physically—believe me, I have been very much involved. This problem has definitely been *my* problem. I have been on the receiving end of many a tearful phone call, "Mom, I can't take it anymore." I have not only felt the extreme pain of my daughter, Roni—I also feel Shae-Lynne's pain. I believe the distance between us has actually kept us closer. It has pushed me to become more involved. I found myself in a room with Shae-Lynne, her mom and dad, and some friends and I realized that I was the main speaker, telling our company, "Shae-Lynne does this, Shae-Lynne does that, etc." I then realized that I have only spent four weeks over the past year with her, yet I know her completely. I thank Roni that she has allowed me to be so involved and has always kept me up-to-date.

This book was written not about one child—it is about all suffering children. All parents will relate to our feelings. This book is a true story; however, we have changed some of the names of the people involved to protect their privacy. You will learn a great deal: firstly, you are not alone, where to get help, what is happening to your child physically, formulas that may help, alternative treatments, how to get answers from your doctor, when an occupational therapist (OT) may help your child and much more.

We share with you the difficulties and obstacles experienced daily and how we found some relief; but we need more answers. This must be a joint project. We will help each other; we have to in order to help our children.

A pediatrician, internist, or neurologist did not write *Life on the Reflux Roller Coaster*, it was written by two women who are trying to make a difference. We cannot let things stay as they are. We cannot keep on doing as we've been doing or we'll keep on getting what we've been getting. In our denial, our children pay the price. Let's get *infant* GERD out of the closet.

After you have read this book you will realize you are not alone. Your child's disease may be a different health issue altogether; however, I think we all feel the same—helpless.

There is help. Your child's welfare is at stake. What could be more important?

As told by Jean McNeil

CHAPTER ONE

OBVIOUSLY, THE BEGINNING

I laid the pregnancy test on the counter beside the sink and stood in the middle of the bathroom staring at the floor. I was waiting for this small plastic stick to tell me my future. As I waited I remember thinking how amazing it was that my whole life might be about to change in an instant. I was scared to look at the results. The seconds went by and my thoughts raced. I so wanted a baby after never really getting over a miscarriage some years earlier. But, was I really ready for this? Can I handle midnight feedings? I do so treasure getting a full ten hours of sleep at night.

There it was, the little blue line. I stood there, motionless, unable to move. I think shock had set in. Michael, my husband, was very comfortable lying on the couch watching his favorite TV show. Should I interrupt now? I wondered. When I finally made my way out to tell him that he was going to be a father, I was surprised at how excited he was and thankfully it put my mind at ease. Of course, we were ready for this. We had been together for about eight years and married for almost three. Yes, it was about time.

As Michael and I talked, I looked at him wondering if our baby would have his dark, wavy hair, or green eyes, maybe his chin or nose. We were both getting excited already.

Then it occurred to me. How do I tell my mom? She's not going to like the idea of being a grandmother. She doesn't like to admit her age. This will really freak her out. My mom eats healthy. She goes to the gym to work out. She is conscious of her appearance, although not overly vain. Although, she once told me, "I will color my hair and wear short skirts until I am a grandmother." Well, Mom….

When I finally got the nerve, I called Mom on October 5th (happens to be my brother Jay's birthday). I was astonished at how excited she was because I knew the Grammy-to-be was thinking, "I'm only mid-40ish, a young mid-

40ish. That's too young to be a grandmother."

Her response made me so very happy. At first she rambled on with so many questions: "When is your due date? How are you feeling? For how long will you continue to work? Have you seen the doctor yet? What hospital are you going to? Do you want a boy or girl? Any names picked out yet? How does Michael feel? Is he excited?" She tends to get carried away and talks a lot. I knew she was as happy as Michael and I were as she continued, "Wow, wow, wow! I am going to be a grandmother! You better take care of yourself." I didn't like being so far away from Mom. It would have been nice if I had been able to share this pregnancy with her. I took pictures of my expanding belly and sent them to her. You can probably imagine how difficult that was to do.

Being nine hundred miles away from your pregnant daughter while she is carrying your grandchild, you think it would be hard to get into this Grammy thing. The miles did not stop my mom. I don't think she could have experienced this pregnancy any more if she had carried the baby herself!

I'll never forget the day she called to tell me about going shopping with Jay for maternity clothes for me. Jay is about six foot, light hair, blue eyes, muscular, a very handsome twenty-five-year-old guy. What a sight it must have been to see this man trotting along behind my mother, the soon-to-be grandmother, to the maternity store and giving his opinion as she stuffed pillows down her pants to try on the maternity clothes. What a couple.

Along with the many trips to the maternity shop, there were the trips to the post office to mail the clothes on nearly a weekly basis. They all knew her by name. You would not have wanted to pay her phone bills either. Remember, the first grandchild was coming. As I said, Mom talks a lot and wanted to be kept up-to-date on how I was feeling.

Mom was spreading the news fast. I couldn't begin to count how many people she told. I think everyone that knew her wanted this new baby to arrive just so she would calm down. I would like to have been there the day I faxed the picture of the ultrasound to her office. She proudly yelled, "Look, everyone, my new grandchild." Did any of you other grammys-to-be do these things? Mom told me that not getting enough sleep from excitement and anticipation of the big day is what makes grandparents look old.

As the weeks and months passed everyone was increasingly excited about the new baby. Knowing that I was due in May and would not be returning to work until the fall, I had our summer plans all set. Picnics by the water, hiking the falls near our house, going to the beach, all with our new little bundle strapped to my belly in the snuggly we would buy. What a great summer we would have.

Michael and I discussed and agreed early on that I would breast-feed. This is by far the best source of nutrition for infants and ours would be the healthiest ever. A whole new life was beginning. I would take exceptionally good care of myself and read all that I could on breast-feeding, childcare and just being a great mom in general.

At nineteen weeks, as Michael and I headed for my ultrasound, we were both so excited. Until now I had not felt any movement, so this was going to be thrilling to finally get some substantial evidence that there was a good reason for my ever-expanding waistline.

As we drove to the appointment, I was remembering the last time I was pregnant (before the miscarriage) and the first ultrasound I had. I drank almost a liter of water about an hour before my appointment, and then I could barely walk down the hall when they called my name because I had to pee so badly. It was really quite painful. I decided at this appointment I would be smart, I would wait until just ten minutes before the ultrasound was scheduled and then drink the water. Boy, was I clever. I thought I had such a great plan until I arrived at the office. As I sat in the parking lot, I realized I had less than ten minutes to drink a liter of water.

Somehow, guzzle after guzzle, I got it down. Then, of course, I had a huge pain in my stomach. I guess I wasn't so smart after all. Michael and I headed down the hall of the hospital where in just a few months we would be leaving as three. It was hard to believe.

The ultrasound technician called us in and began dumping gobs of cold clear jelly on my stomach. As she moved the wand around, an image began to appear. Tears escaped my eyes as I saw our baby for the first time. I never expected the images to be so clear. The baby's whole body was right there on the screen. I did not want this moment to end. I studied every inch as if to burn the image into my memory. Two little feet, two little legs, tiny little bum, back and belly, two arms and hands, shoulders, head and face. We counted the fingers, ten, perfect. We saw the whole face, eyes, nose, and mouth. Wow! The only thing we couldn't see was whether it was a boy or girl.

The baby kicked, rolled, flipped, and moved about like crazy. I was amazed at the amount of activity and I wasn't feeling any of it. Each fist was positioned by each ear and at one point the little fist opened up and seemed to wave at us. I will always treasure this moment. Michael and I drove home in almost complete silence, each of us feeling so much love for this beautiful new life and replaying the ultrasound in our minds.

Month after month together Michael and I went for my routine checkups. Everything was normal and going fine. It was great having Michael so involved and supportive. He came with me to every checkup. Now at the twenty-eight-week mark we were on our way to another checkup. I felt so huge I could not imagine going another twelve weeks. I already looked like a beached whale and gave up putting on shoes unless they slipped on. It was hard to believe that I could get any bigger. Being only about five feet tall, I had decided that I am too short to be pregnant. There's simply no place for the baby to go but out.

My excitement about the pregnancy was being overshadowed by extreme nausea. I grudgingly took Diclectin, a drug prescribed to help eliminate excessive vomiting during pregnancy. If I didn't take the medicine I'd be throwing up all day. This was more than morning sickness. I couldn't eat anything at all without it coming back up and even if I didn't eat I felt sick all day.

At this checkup there was nothing overly eventful to report to my obstetrician, Dr. Elizabeth Ruth. I told her I still had to take the Diclectin and that concerned me. I didn't like the idea of taking medication when I was pregnant. Every couple of weeks I would try to go a day without the medication and the outcome was always the same. I just couldn't keep anything down. I remember one night being so thirsty I desperately wanted a glass of water but really didn't feel like throwing up again, so opted for ice cubes. Within ten minutes I was even throwing up the ice cubes.

Dr. Ruth explained to me that it was all right if I had to take the Diclectin the entire nine months. It's perfectly safe and many women have to take it throughout their whole pregnancy.

Dr. Ruth started by listening to the heartbeat. I love this part: "145bpm—perfect." She then got out her tape to measure my belly. "Hmmm," she muttered under her breath. "A little large."

"No kidding," I laughed. She decided to do a pelvic exam and told me I was partly effaced. Apparently this happens shortly before labor. It is not supposed to happen this early.

She explained that the baby might just be big but she thought I had extra amniotic fluid, which could cause premature labor. Another ultrasound was scheduled the following week, just to make sure. Dr. Ruth would not be available then; however, her partner would be there and we would see him if the technician felt there was a concern.

I was looking forward to having another ultrasound; the first was so thrilling. Unfortunately, this time the baby was too big, the images weren't as clear and there wasn't as much movement. The ultrasound technician wouldn't tell us much of anything, but we didn't have to wait to see the obstetrician. We were sent right home. I felt relief, believing everything must have been fine. A couple of weeks passed and my doctor's secretary called me to schedule an appointment for an early checkup the following week.

I was thirty-two weeks along when we went back to see Dr. Ruth. It was quite a drive, well over an hour; however, Dr. Ruth was the type of doctor you didn't mind driving any distance to see. She made me feel very comfortable and overall I just liked her.

"Well, it looks as if my suspicion was accurate. You do, in fact, have extra amniotic fluid," Dr. Ruth began.

"Okay, so now what? What exactly does this mean?" I questioned, not understanding the problem completely.

"Well...." She went on, "The excessive fluid can fool your body into believing you are further along than you actually are and this could cause you to go into labor a couple weeks early. I'd like to do another exam to see if you have progressed since the last visit." She helped me out of the chair and we moved towards the examination bed and she drew the curtain.

I really wasn't seeing a big problem with going into labor a couple weeks early. Thirty-eight weeks sounded just find to me.

As I prepared for the exam, Dr. Ruth continued. "I want you to take it easy for the next few weeks." As she came around the corner of the curtain and began her exam, I wondered, what did she mean "take it easy"?

"Hmmm," mumbling to herself and looking a bit more alarmed now, "oh yes, you've already started to dilate."

What? I thought. This may be my first baby but I knew enough to know that to dilate means you go into labor! I felt panic for a moment but was still very much in denial. Certainly *I* won't have any complications; that happens to other people. I was sure she was exaggerating.

"What do you mean I've started to dilate? But, I'm not in labor." I was slightly puzzled and sat waiting for a quick answer to explain all this away.

"Yes, but the labor could start any time now. I want you to go home and rest from now on."

"What do you mean rest?" I wanted to make sure we were all perfectly clear on Dr. Ruth's instructions. I was picturing the dirty dishes at home sitting in the sink and I was really looking for an excuse to get out of doing them. What better way to get Michael to do them than for the doctor to confirm that I couldn't? "You mean no housework until after the baby is born?" I grinned in a disbelieving manner.

"That's right, no dishes, no cleaning…" She looked over at Michael who appeared to be more concerned than I was at this point. "And definitely, no vacuuming." Dr. Ruth really stressed that. "Go straight home and lay down."

"Hehe," I giggled to Michael, "wait until I tell Janet tomorrow at work that she has to do the vacuuming from now on." Janet and I worked together in the office of a local factory. She was my boss, the office manager, and I had been hired to do the bookkeeping. It was just the two of us and so I would do some light tidying up when it was needed, including vacuuming the floor once a week or so.

"I don't think you should be going back to work," Michael commented. He seemed annoyed that I didn't appear to be taking this seriously.

"Of course I can go to work," I said, looking toward Dr. Ruth for reassurance, "all I do is sit at my desk all day."

"No, Roni, you cannot go back to work. I told you, you have to rest," she retorted.

Certainly, Dr. Ruth did not understand. I had too much to do. I was in the middle of converting all the books, currently still being done on paper, to the computer system. How was I supposed to train someone to do my job when I was in the middle of that mess? Never mind that we didn't even have a replacement in mind yet.

After explaining my predicament, I began an attempt at bartering for more time at work.

"Well, I have to go in for one more week. I have to do at least that. I mean it's only a desk job. I sit all day. That's not exerting." Surely, now she would understand.

"I don't think you realize the seriousness of this situation, Roni." Dr. Ruth, although usually quiet and soft-spoken, seemed to be losing her patience with me. "You could go into labor any minute and the baby is not ready to be born yet. The lungs are one of the last things to form and if the baby were born now, they wouldn't be fully developed yet. Your baby would almost certainly need to be put on a ventilator for the first few weeks and could end up with long-term respiratory problems. Sitting is just as bad as standing. You need to remain flat—to fight gravity—keep horizontal. I mean, complete bed rest. This is serious," she concluded and seemed rather angry that I was not listening.

We left the office and I cried the entire hour and a half drive home. How was I going to tell Janet? I was so concerned about leaving my job before a replacement had been found and before I finished everything I needed to. How was Janet going to get everything done alone? I left work for my appointment that day with a hundred things left to do at the office and now with no notice, I couldn't go back. I couldn't even train my replacement. I didn't even have a replacement yet. I felt awful.

As I look back I cannot believe how naive I was. Even then, when put on complete bed rest, never once did I expect to have anything but a perfectly healthy baby. Maybe it was just easier to worry about work than the possibility of a premature baby.

I had things to do; I couldn't go on bed rest. But I had to, doctor's orders, and so I did. I was so very lucky Verne my *other* mom took very good care of me. I had known her since I was fourteen when Mom, Jay and I first rented an apartment from her. It was a tough time for all of us. Mom and Dad had just separated. Being teenagers at the time, Jay and I were not the easiest people to get along with. Somehow, Verne saw through that and we became very close. During the few years that we lived there we began to feel like a family. Now, here she was years later giving up her time for me. She made me lunches, did laundry, washed the dishes and any other chores that needed to be done. Verne had four kids of her own and a very busy schedule. I don't know what I would have done without her. I was very glad every time she stopped by to help out or even to just visit.

I had to go for weekly checkups and week after week Michael and I went and heard, "You're one centimeter…it may happen anytime; you're two centimeters…it may happen anytime, you're three centimeters…" and so on. Thirty-four weeks and counting….

CHAPTER TWO

MY BABY WON'T EAT

My thirty-four-week mark came and went without event, and finally at thirty-nine weeks on a Tuesday our beautiful (proud mom talking) little girl was born. Thank God, we made it this far! An even seven pounds with the longest, thickest, black hair I had ever seen on a newborn. Our beautiful little miracle, our daughter Shae-Lynne, had arrived. Michael and I had been discussing baby names the past few months. He heard of the name Shae and liked that. I wasn't thrilled with it. I wanted to name her Brooke. One day while searching a baby name book I came across the name Shae-Lynne, so we compromised and decided on Shae-Lynne Brooke.

Immediately following the delivery, the nurses cleaned Shae-Lynne, put her in a crib and left her. Before I knew what was going on, every nurse in the room was running in a different direction. Another doctor came in and started a second intravenous in my arm and my obstetrician was calling for blood. I didn't like knowing that Shae-Lynne was spending her first few minutes of life lying alone. She seemed content, but I felt badly and noticed Michael in the opposite corner. I asked him to pick her up but I think he was nervous. Apparently I was hemorrhaging and everyone was trying to get that under control. Michael decided he didn't want to be in the way so he headed out to the cell phone in the car to call everyone.

He called his mom first. Granny Dorothy was thrilled and couldn't wait for us to get home so she could see Shae-Lynne. Next, he called my mom—she was beside herself and already planning a trip here. She and Jay would drive here from Boston after work on Friday. Michael told her I would call her tomorrow or the next day when I was feeling better.

* * *

Because I had hemorrhaged so badly, it was well over an hour, maybe two, before I was allowed to hold and nurse Shae-Lynne. The first attempt at nursing didn't go well. She didn't appear to be the least bit hungry. The nurses were concerned that I rest, and since Shae-Lynne would not eat anyway, I reluctantly agreed to let them take her to the nursery. I asked to be awakened the second she woke up. I lay awake all night waiting for the nurses. I stared endlessly at the wall and the ceiling. All the *Sesame Street* characters kept me company that evening. They seemed to come alive. I thought Big Bird was smiling at me—okay, so maybe I was tired, or lost a little too much blood. I knew every detail of the room. I heard every noise during the quiet night as most moms and babies slept. Every time I heard footsteps I grew excited, as I was sure they were coming with Shae-Lynne.

It was nine a.m. when a nurse finally walked into the room to check on me. "Good morning. How did you sleep?" she asked as she moved across the room towards my bed.

"I didn't. Where is my daughter?" I said abruptly. I was sure since they had not brought her to me through the night they must have given her a bottle even though they promised not to. They had to have given her something. Babies don't sleep through the night.

"Oh, don't worry about her. She's still sleeping." The nurse seemed very nice but I was slightly frustrated that no one thought perhaps I may want to see my new baby and bring her to me, sleeping or not.

"Why didn't anyone bring her to me through the night? I'm supposed to be nursing her and I lay awake all night waiting for her."

"Well, you needed your rest and she's been sleeping all night so we didn't want to wake either of you." The nurse was not concerned at all that Shae-Lynne hadn't woken since she fell asleep shortly after her birth twelve hours earlier.

"She hasn't woken up at all?" I repeated.

The nurse must have sensed the fear in my voice because she began to reassure me. "No, but don't worry. It's very common and you know she's had a busy day. Besides, the drug you were given in the epidural can make some babies sleepy. She'll come around, she's been through a lot for such a tiny thing."

Okay, made sense to me, she has, after all, seen a lot more newborns than I have. "But I really want to see her. Can't she stay in the room with me?" I was getting desperate.

"Are you sure you don't want to get some rest?" she replied, still trying to be helpful.

"No, I can't sleep without her here anyway."

"All right, I'll bring her right in." She left the room.

A few minutes later the same nurse wheeled in the crib with a still sleeping Shae-Lynne. Wow, she was so beautiful she took my breath away! "Can I hold her?"

"Well, since she is still sleeping I'm going to go and I will let you rest awhile," she said, as she passed me Shae-Lynne. "Use the buzzer to call me when she wakes and we'll get started on nursing." With that said she left again.

I lay there close to an hour just holding and staring at Shae-Lynne. I knew I needed sleep but couldn't make myself close my eyes. Finally, she started to wake so I buzzed for the nurse to make sure the nursing went well.

First Shae-Lynne did not seem interested and wouldn't latch on properly. Then eventually when we got her latched she wouldn't suck. She was still and drifted back to sleep. UGH! It had been the same the first time I had tried to nurse her. I was so worried. *She has to eat.* She *must* be hungry by now.

The nurse and I worked for a while longer trying to get Shae-Lynne to wake up and actually eat something but to no avail. I had read enough about nursing to know it's very important to get the nursing established as early after birth as possible and time was not on my side at this point. I felt tears in my eyes.

The nurse sensed what I was feeling. "It's okay, the effects of the epidural could last for a couple days. We'll just get you pumping to build up your milk until Shae-Lynne comes around." The nurse was so sure of herself. It put me at ease as she went to get the breast pump.

The feeding schedule was set at every three hours. So, three hours later the nurse came back and we tried again. Again, Shae-Lynne would not eat. She still wouldn't even wake up. Same response from the nurses, "It's okay, just keep pumping. She doesn't know what she is supposed to do, this eating thing is new to her, give her time to adjust." The pump was permanently parked beside my bed and after twenty minutes of trying to get Shae-Lynne to eat anything at all, I was back to expressing twenty minutes per side.

I called my mother to let her know we were both doing well and to fill her in with more details. I told her I was a bit worried, as Shae-Lynne didn't seem to want to eat and slept all the time.

Mom responded, "Roni, what do you mean she won't eat? I never heard of such a thing. Babies always eat. That's what babies do."

I was sure she thought I was overreacting, as did the nurses. I was to hear this same line over and over from so many people as Shae-Lynne continued her refusal to eat.

The epidural excuse was wearing thin after a few days. Now I heard that Shae-Lynne didn't have the energy to eat because she hadn't eaten in so long. Nursing is hard work for babies. Give her a little formula, build up her strength, and then she will take right off with nursing. I knew that was a big mistake. I knew if I started formula Shae-Lynne would not be hungry enough to build up my already waning milk supply. Instinct told me it was wrong to supplement with formula but I felt there was no choice. We had to try something. Shae-Lynne needed help.

We tried Similac in a one-ounce medicine cup. She kept her mouth closed. The nurse tried again by opening her mouth and pouring it in. It dribbled out. UGH! The frustration. Why won't she eat? Every three hours I had to nurse, try to get formula into her, and then express my milk with a breast pump. By the time I had finished one feeding, it was time for the next. Shae-Lynne was still not getting the nutrition she needed. Something was wrong.

When Shae-Lynne was sleeping I would spend every second staring at her. Her beauty struck me. She was so perfect. How could anything be wrong? I would lay awake with my eyes burning from exhaustion knowing I should be sleeping and yet I rarely could. I couldn't take my eyes off her, nor could I have imagined feeling this much love. And yet, I had a nagging sense of worry.

About the third day after Shae-Lynne was born I had started asking when we could be released. Our doctor didn't want us to leave the hospital until the nursing was well established and Shae-Lynne was back to her birth weight. That evening after Michael had gone home and I finished trying to nurse Shae-Lynne I put her to bed and proceeded with my routine of sitting on the bed while crying and pumping. I felt horrible. When was this going to end? I wanted Shae-Lynne to eat and my milk production to increase more than I had ever wanted anything in my life. I was doing everything I could to make it happen but it just wasn't good enough.

As I sat alone with my tears, a nurse popped her head in to check on me.

"Hi there, how's it going?" she asked. But with one look at me she didn't have to wait for an answer. She came in and sat on the bed beside me. All the nurses were trying to be helpful—I know they wanted this to work almost as much as I did. I especially liked this particular nurse. She was quite familiar with what had been going on with Shae-Lynne and knew immediately why I was crying.

"Oh, Roni, I wish there was something more I could do to help," she began as she gently patted my leg.

I was crying so hard I couldn't even respond. I've always been a private person and I hated being so vulnerable and having people see me like this.

I began to put the breast pump away and try to compose myself, as she continued. "You know, I was just talking with the other nurses and everyone was commenting on how strong you have been the past few days." That got a chuckle out of me. She continued, "We all really admire your dedication and think you have given nursing more of an effort than just about anyone we've seen. Your persistence is great, but maybe it's time to think about letting it go. You know millions of babies have grown up on formula and they do just fine. No one here is going to think any less of you or think you are a quitter if you give up on it, and you shouldn't either. No one wants you to feel pressured into continuing."

With that I was crying even harder. This was the first time that giving up had entered my mind. Did she really think this wasn't going to work for us?

Noticing her comments had not helped, she moved closer to me to give me a hug. After a moment she moved back and continued, "You have lasted longer and tried harder to make this work than anyone expects and we are all behind you whatever you decide. We'll continue to do anything we can to help if you decide to keep trying to breast-feed, but just the fact that Shae-Lynne took some breast milk is great and you shouldn't feel guilty about any of this."

My stomach was sick and my chest hurt just thinking about it. It wasn't supposed to be this hard. The entire time she sat and spoke, I was praying this would all go away, imagining myself somewhere else—anywhere other than with a new baby that wouldn't eat and not having to listen to her speak about quitting something so important. "I'll give you a few minutes alone to think things over. I'll come back later and you can let me know what you decide." She tapped my leg again and I nodded. She turned to walk out and as soon as the door closed behind her, I cried even harder. Give up? Is that what she wanted me to do? Apparently she didn't know me very well. Giving up was simply not an option.

While I was pregnant, I read about and heard many stories of women who had tried to breast-feed and for different reasons were unable to do so. They just gave up. Every time I heard that, I judged them and couldn't understand how they could simply give up on something so incredibly important. I knew I would make it work. I wouldn't be one of *those* women. Now, as I was faced with this decision myself, I couldn't help but notice the irony. I thought so little of those who had given up and couldn't do it. Part of me thought this was some sort of cosmic lesson I needed to learn and because of my arrogance, I was being made to eat a little crow. I had new respect for what mothers who could not breast-feed experienced.

Cosmic lesson or not, I was not a quitter. I dried my tears, pulled myself together and felt a renewed sense of strength. I felt as though I needed this nurse. She helped me find the courage and resiliency that I thought had left me.

For four days and nights, I was nursing every three hours and then pumping to build up a milk supply for a child who wasn't keeping up her end of nature's supply-and-demand principle. Shae-Lynne had lost weight as all babies do when they are first born, but she just wasn't gaining it back. I was reassured she was fine.

To add to our difficulties, it was taking longer than it should have for my milk to come in. I would spend every day crying, nursing, pumping and crying some more. This was my fault and I felt so awful. I knew I was such a failure. If only this beautiful little girl had been born to someone who wasn't so useless. I couldn't do pregnancy right. I couldn't do labor right. Now I couldn't do this right. I hated myself and I hated my body for betraying me and for betraying Shae-Lynne.

Obviously, the nurses couldn't blame me out loud. They had a number of other theories: Shae-Lynne's lack of interest, the drug I was given to stop the hemorrhaging, the stress on my body from the hemorrhage, stress in general, not eating enough, and not drinking enough…you name it. It didn't matter because I knew the truth. I knew what they were thinking, because I was thinking it too. I was useless.

Another theory was that Shae-Lynne was not latching on properly which could cause poor milk production. The biggest problem women have with nursing is mastering the elusive latch. Every nurse and lactation consultant in the hospital came to watch me nurse (talk about lack of privacy, and my dignity had long since jumped ship). It was agreed, when I managed to keep Shae-Lynne awake, that the latching technique had been mastered. Latching was not the problem.

After four days I convinced the doctor to let us go home on the basis that we would go for a daily weigh in at our local hospital until Shae-Lynne started gaining weight. I was sure that if we could just go home things would settle down. Stress was our whole problem. We needed to go home and relax.

* * *

I guess Mom knew she was needed. After working all day, she and Jay were headed this way. They drove all night (approximately a fourteen-hour drive) and got lost in Maine. I didn't believe it. This is a trip they have both done more times than you would believe. Was it the excitement or a need for glasses? She is a grandmother now. They arrived at the hospital at six thirty a.m. and as I was trying to sleep, they sneaked into our room. I was so happy to see them and the time of day didn't matter.

You could see the love in her eyes as my mom said, "There's Shae-Lynne. Look at her, so tiny, so beautiful. Soooooo much hair. Look at her. She's perfect. Simply perfect."

She paused only briefly as she leaned over, picked Shae-Lynne up and kissed her forehead. She continued, "I am finally holding her, a precious little angel. A gift from God."

After hugs and kisses and a bit of catching up, I explained further the events of the previous days. Shae-Lynne was not eating and I was not producing breast milk, as I should. Her response was, "Roni, no wonder, you just went through a complicated delivery and to think they are giving Tylenol with codeine to someone breast-feeding! That stuff puts me to sleep." That made sense to me so I stopped taking the Tylenol with codeine. I really wasn't in much pain anyway.

It was finally time to get ready to go home. We were all busy. I was getting Shae-Lynne ready while Michael and Mom were packing up our things. We forget about Jay for a minute until we heard laughter outside our room. A new father with his three children walking past our room noticed Jay asleep on my bed. It must have seemed odd to them to see a big guy snoring in bed in the maternity ward. We all left the hospital that day so happy. Michael and I had our new little baby and our family was all together.

* * *

I was glad Mom came up; I needed her support. It was great to see Jay again also, as he is my only brother. There is only a year between us and we've always been very close. Mom had been telling me about the wonderful girl he had started dating. Karen would be flying up this weekend and I was looking forward to meeting her. Now we would meet under these rather stressful circumstances. Karen definitely saw the worst. Thankfully, as soon as I met her, I liked her a lot. I felt very comfortable with her and didn't feel like I had to be a hostess or pretend everything was wonderful while she was there. I knew she was the one for Jay. I was already planning; *they* would be Shae-Lynne's Godparents. I was so happy for my brother.

I thought that once we were home, things would be better. Unfortunately, they were not. Shae-Lynne still wasn't eating. Not only would she not eat, she wouldn't stay awake to eat. Nothing we seemed to do would keep her awake. Why was she sleeping so much? We continued the daily weigh in at the local hospital and the pressure from that was killing me. With every feeding I was consumed with what the scale was going to say the next day. Whether she lost weight, maintained her weight or had simply not gained as much as they thought she should, I heard, "You have to be more aggressive. Just relax, she senses your stress." At every feeding I was undressing Shae-Lynne and feeding her diapered only, the purpose being to keep her somewhat cool and uncomfortable so she would stay awake and hopefully eat. I was told to wipe her forehead with a cool, damp cloth (reasoning as above), tickle her feet, rub her head (from the forehead back as the other way may put her to sleep), massage her cheek, roll the nipple around in her mouth, rub her tongue, inner cheek and the roof of her mouth with gentle pressure and stroke underneath her chin with my fingers. Nothing worked. Shae-Lynne still chose sleeping over eating.

She didn't seem to get hungry, but why? Usually an infant wakes when they are hungry. Shae-Lynne wouldn't wake. At the age of one week I had to set the alarm through the night to wake and feed her. One night I had forgotten to set the alarm and she slept over seven hours having only one half-ounce of breast milk in her stomach. The only reason she woke then was that I happened to wake up. Shae-Lynne may have been our first child; however, I knew what we were experiencing simply wasn't normal infant behavior. We asked ourselves so many questions but there didn't seem to be any answers. We knew she had to eat. How else was she to gain weight? We knew that only too well as we went each day to the hospital for her weigh in. Each day we were told to get her to eat, as if we didn't already know that! The next day, the same thing, Shae-Lynne would not eat. Shae-Lynne would not wake up. Day after day nothing changed. Shae-Lynne was more determined not to eat. We were more determined that she must.

41

* * *

Beep, beep, beep. The sharp piercing beep of the alarm wakes me abruptly. I wonder how long I'd been asleep as I roll over to shut off the alarm. I'm not really awake and not sure what time of day it is. I must have been extremely tired because I feel like I've been asleep for a year. I look at the clock. It's three a.m. Rubbing my eyes I begin to regain my senses and realize I've slept only about half an hour. It was almost 2:30 a.m. when I crawled into bed after the last feeding.

"Please, please, eat. Please, please, please, *just eat something this time,*" I mutter over and over again as I crawl out of bed and head for Shae-Lynne's cradle. She is, of course, sleeping as I look in at her and reach to pick her up. We head toward the living room and in preparation for this feed I begin to talk to her, hoping to wake her.

"Okay, angel, wake up for Mommy. Time to wake up, sweetie. Shae-Lynne, Shae-Lynne. Come on Shae, time to eat, honey." *Yeah, this is not working.* I make a pit stop in the bathroom to get a cool, wet face cloth—all the while thinking, this is crazy.

We settle in on the couch and the struggle begins. I wipe her forehead and the top of her head with the cold, wet cloth. This gets Shae-Lynne's attention and see begins to wake. She latches for me and I get excited. I sit quietly, listening and watching for the suck, suck, swallow motions that I've been trained to watch for. She starts dozing off again. I wipe her down once more with the cool cloth. It's not working, so I have to undress her. Now she seems to be awake and we start all over, this time on the other side, as it's already been twenty minutes. She finally starts to eat some and I'm so relieved. I glance toward the clock to time how long she is on this side before I must break out the bottle. It's less than two minutes and she's asleep yet again. UGH! I want to scream. I decide to change her bum, maybe that will wake her. She's so darn cute, wiggling and squirming. She is bright eyed and bushy tailed now, so it's back to the couch and the breast. She's awake, she's latched but she's just not sucking. *What a nightmare.* She's got to be hungry, she only took half an ounce at her last feeding and I can hear her little belly growling. Next, I try rubbing her cheek, hoping to get her to suck—this is pulling from the bag of tricks suggested by her nurses. This dance continues for fifteen minutes more. Finally, I give up and get the bottle out. The same routine begins with the bottle. Forty-five minutes later and I have only managed to get her to take a half ounce. I decide to give up.

As I dress Shae-Lynne, I start to cry—again. It's now almost four-thirty a.m. She's scheduled to be fed again at six. Of course, there is no way to know how much breast milk she got. Based on how much (or how little, I should say) I've been pumping and how little I heard her actually swallow, I suspect it's no more than a half ounce. That puts her total intake, at this feed, to be one ounce. Actually, this was not a bad feed. I know it's not enough and think about the impending weigh in tomorrow, I mean, today. I feel so guilty for giving up but I know we can't sit here all night continuing like this, so I put her back to bed. I then get out the breast pump, express each side for fifteen minutes. Finally, I clean the pump before crawling back to bed. It is now shortly after five a.m. We did all right this time; I have close to one hour before Shae-Lynne is to be fed again.

* * *

It's hard to believe how fast an hour can pass. There goes the alarm again: beep, beep, beep; it's six a.m. We start all over.

I still wasn't producing enough breast milk. Everyone kept telling me stress was probably a big factor and that I needed to relax. I don't know how anyone expected that to happen with the way things were going. Every moment of the day and night was spent trying to feed Shae-Lynne. I had no time to myself. I was pumping constantly although I did not have an ounce of strength left. I guess it is a case of supply and demand. If the child is not demanding, the body is not going to produce. Hence, continue to pump. Unfortunately, pumping is not as effective as nursing and it just wasn't helping.

If only she would eat, *we* wouldn't have to go through all this. (Note: "we" wouldn't have to go through all this. Actually, the bottom line is the new mother is the one producing the breast milk, or should I say trying to.) But Michael and Mom were also very much affected by watching all this. It is agonizing when you want to help, but there is nothing you can do. We all have stories to tell our children when they are grown. My favorite will be when Michael, the proud dad, told everyone, "We were up all night breast-feeding." Oh, *we* were—were *we*?

Nearly two horrific weeks had passed. Shae-Lynne was not gaining nearly what she should have and was not even back to her birth weight. It was heartbreaking to watch our child starve herself. Not knowing why was the worst part. Although no one said it out loud, I sensed people were thinking that we were doing something wrong. I sensed them thinking it because part of me was thinking it too. Of course, we heard every suggestion: "Why don't you just force her" or "Wait until she gets hungry, just forget the schedule" or "I'd do this" or "Have you tried?" I knew the suggestions were meant to be helpful, but they left me feeling more inadequate, if that were possible.

My energy was draining each day and with each feeding and I would cry, "I can't keep doing this…I can't do this anymore!" I had never considered myself to be overly emotional and certainly was not the type to cry, especially in front of anyone. In fact before Shae-Lynne, I can't remember the last time I did cry. However, I was making up for it now. Michael was getting angry and frustrated, unable to show his pain. My mom would jump in and cuddle Shae-Lynne, praying and whispering in her ear, "Healing, joy, peace and love." Love is always the answer, isn't it? Love will fix this.

This was to be a happy time. We daydreamed, we waited and we planned. It wasn't supposed to be like this.

We didn't think it could get any worse. It did. The night before Mom and Jay were to go home, Shae-Lynne started throwing up. She choked and gagged so forcefully, it was frightening. She looked up at me with fear and confusion in her eyes, almost begging me to make it stop. Again, I start to cry. I stare at the floor and the pool of formula that I had just sweated blood to get into her and now it was just a big mess to clean up. Shaking my head in disbelief, I think, *what next?*

* * *

It was Monday night; tomorrow Shae-Lynne would be two weeks old. We had an exceptionally bad day; she took only four ounces (120 mls) all day and had thrown up most of it. I couldn't take this anymore, so I called our family doctor. However, Dr. Tardanico was on call that evening.

Sadly Mom and Jay had to head for home and left shortly before our doctor's appointment.

I was prepared as we headed over to see Dr. Tardanico. I made notes of what Shae-Lynne had taken in all day and how often she had vomited. I thought having it on paper for him to see would make him understand I was not exaggerating. As we waited to see him I told myself to be strong and not to cry.

"So, how's it going?" he asked as he walked in the door with a friendly smile.

I burst into tears; so much for being strong. "Please, you have to do something to make Shae-Lynne eat. I have tried everything—she simply will not eat. She won't wake up and now she has also started to throw up. This is not anything I am doing. Please, don't tell me to be more aggressive! You have to do something to help," I pleaded. I had to make him understand I wasn't an idiot first-time mother that didn't know what to do. I knew there was something wrong and if only I could make him understand, then he would be able to fix this.

"Okay, okay, calm down," he began as he passed me a tissue. "What has Shae-Lynne eaten today?"

I passed my notes with her intake and the vomiting that she had done for the day, as I explained what feeding her (or rather trying to) was really like. He listened intently and began to examine and weigh her as I spoke.

"Yes, I agree, there is something going on here. I'm going to see if I can get a hold of Dr. Andrews, a pediatrician in Sydney, to see if he should see her." With that he left the room to make the call. Sydney, the closest city to us, had a much larger hospital than the small town we lived in and, therefore, Dr. Tardanico felt that Dr. Andrews would be better equipped to help Shae-Lynne.

By this time, I was hysterical as this was the first confirmation that something was actually wrong with our little girl and I didn't feel I could cope with that.

Dr. Tardanico came back into the room after what seemed an eternity and said, "Dr Andrews does feel that Shae-Lynne needs to be looked at and he is arranging to have her admitted to the Neonatal Intensive Care Unit (NICU). He'll be waiting for you."

It felt as though a truck had just hit me. "You mean right now?" I managed between sobs.

"Yes, go home now and pack a few things. You will probably be there a few days. Dr. Andrews is concerned that Shae-Lynne may be dehydrated and need an IV." Dr. Tardanico patted my arm and passed me more tissue. "Don't worry," he continued, "they are used to babies with feeding problems. They'll figure out what's going on," he said with a reassuring smile.

For a brief moment, while at home packing to leave for Sydney, we felt somewhat relieved that the doctors were finally beginning to acknowledge that something was wrong. Then it suddenly hit me; something is really wrong with our beautiful little girl! I cried and my body trembled in fear. This hospital was over an hour's drive away. This night the drive seemed to take much longer. I was terrified. Michael seemed stronger, but I knew he was just better at hiding his fear and pain.

When we arrived at the hospital and met Dr. Andrews, he assured us they would find the problem. However, he warned that it could take some time. It was a comfort to meet him. He's a tall and somewhat handsome man and his caring nature had a calming effect on us. He made us feel as though we were important and really did matter.

Dr. Andrews ordered many tests, including the usual blood count, electrolytes, oxygen saturation, electrocardiogram (ECG/EKG), chest x-ray, and electroencephalogram (EEG). The ECG/EKG is an electrical recording of the heart. The EEG is a brain wave test. They also did an ultrasound on Shae-Lynne's heart since babies with heart problems usually sleep through feeds, because they do not have enough energy to eat. Dr. Andrews also heard a murmur in her heart so the test was sent to Children's Hospital for a second opinion, which eventually turned out fine. My gut feeling was telling me Shae-Lynne did not have a heart problem. She didn't seem to exhibit the symptoms that Dr. Andrews had described.

We spent two weeks in NICU waiting and watching as many tests were performed. Maybe it could be this…maybe that…. Each time we prepared ourselves for the worst and learned that each and every test was normal. We started to relax as some of the more serious things were ruled out. However, we still had the problem of no diagnosis. The entire time I had been telling the nurses, Dr. Andrews and the neonatologist that Shae-Lynne was throwing up too much. It was dismissed as overreacting. "Some babies are just pukers…some babies are just spitters…don't worry, it's never as much as it seems."

Not once during this hospital stay did the doctors try to find out why she was vomiting and gagging. Not once did it occur to them that if they found out why she was vomiting, they would figure out why Shae-Lynne was not eating.

It was a very difficult time in the hospital. I never left it the entire time Shae-Lynne was there. I was alone every day, all day with Shae-Lynne. Michael had to work each day. If he wanted to see Shae-Lynne and me (which he did), he had to do the two-hour plus drive each night. This made it a very long day. We were both beyond exhausted.

Watching Shae-Lynne throw up was definitely the hardest part. First there would be a cough or two, and then her mouth would wiggle a little. You knew it was coming. Time to quickly grab a towel. Most of the time we could even hear it coming up. We could almost track the acid, stomach juices and formula as it moved up Shae-Lynne's esophagus and into her throat. With the first gag, her mouth would open and nothing would come up. Her eyes watered. It didn't always come all the way up, just far enough to make her gag. I would see it come just to the back of her throat, then go back down, knowing with each movement up and down it would burn her tiny throat and esophagus. She would scream in pain and fright with those blue eyes staring up into mine with terror and begging, "Mommy, make it stop!" I felt so helpless. There would be more screaming and another gag. Shae-Lynne's face would turn beet red as a ball of thick mucous gushed out of her mouth and sometimes even her nose at the same time. She would try to scream again but her screams would be cut off as her airway became blocked with mucous. Shae-Lynne would look at me again as she gasped for air. "Mommy, what's happening?" Gag after endless gag for minutes at a time brought up more and more mucous. Her face would become even redder. Tears poured down her cheeks and her heart beat almost out of her chest. I have been through this so often, I see it in my sleep. It does not get any easier for her or for us.

* * *

In lieu of a diagnosis, the doctors had labeled Shae-Lynne *Failure to Thrive* (FTT). *What in the world was failure to thrive?* I kept thinking. Talk about making a first-time mom feel like a complete failure. I had to know more about failure to thrive. What is it? What causes it? What do you do to correct it? I had to have answers so I called Mom again. She went to her local library, did some research and faxed her research to me at the hospital.

The term *Failure to Thrive (FTT)* is used to describe a cluster of symptoms. It is not a specific disease. It refers to a lack of proper growth or development and is usually applied to children through age two. FTT is caused by a variety of circumstances. Most infants lose a small amount of weight shortly after they are born but within a few days they should begin to gain weight at a consistent rate. If the baby continues losing weight, or does not gain as anticipated, then it is labeled failure to thrive.

Non-organic FTT (NOFTT) occurs when the baby is not receiving enough food due to parental neglect, economic conditions, or perhaps psycho-social problems. This is an otherwise healthy baby with nothing medically wrong. There is an external cause of the baby's FTT (e.g., a baby being neglected by their parents may become depressed and exhibit poor appetite). This is the most common cause of FTT.

Conversely, organic FTT (OFTT) is caused by an internal health problem. The organs involved in digestion and absorption of food may be malformed or incomplete, making the baby unable to digest its food properly.

Was I getting paranoid or what? According to this definition of FTT, either I was a rotten, unfit mother, or there was something very wrong with my little girl. I was screaming inside.

After the second week in the hospital, Shae-Lynne finally started to wake a little and even accepted a bit of food. It was still a fight to get her to eat and she still wasn't eating anywhere near what an infant her age should be eating. She would take about one-half ounce (15 mls) and not want anymore. At least she was a bit more alert and that was encouraging.

Shae-Lynne was eating so poorly that her neonatologist and Dr. Andrews decided to fortify her formula with extra calories. They increased it from the normal twenty calories per ounce to twenty-four. With this adjustment Shae-Lynne had one to two mediocre weight gains and she was then released on home passes. This meant Shae-Lynne was still a patient and needed to check into the hospital every twenty-four hours. We made the two-hour plus drive to the hospital daily.

* * *

I was convinced that Shae-Lynne needed a new formula. The more I watched her the more I noticed she did much better with the breast milk. It was a little easier to get her to drink it and she really only threw up once. Another time she took a record three ounces (90 mls). I knew it must be due to the breast milk. This added to my guilt since I could not produce enough. My mom insisted that allergies (our family has a history of being sensitive to things) could be the cause of all this. We had read portions of *Is This Your Child* by Dr. Doris Rapp. This exceptional book led the way in explaining how food allergies may affect our health. Now I had to convince Shae-Lynne's doctors to switch her formula.

Eventually the neonatologist did agree to switch to Isomil, which is a soy-based formula. Shae-Lynne seemed to do well on it for about a week until she started to throw up after each feeding. Time to switch again, I thought. Her doctors were not as eager to keep switching formulas. They argued that she needed time to adjust to a new one. I disagreed and insisted on switching. After much persuasion, I convinced them to listen to me. Maybe they listened just to keep me quiet more than anything. I thought there had to be a formula out there that Shae-Lynne could tolerate as well as she did the breast milk. Similac LF was the next try. It's similar to Similac except that it's free of lactose. Shae-Lynne had other plans though and wouldn't take it. She screamed whenever I put it near her. It amazed me how tiny she was and yet she knew what she wanted, or rather, didn't want. We then switched to Carnation Good Start. Good Start is a milk-based formula that has partly broken down protein molecules for easy digestion. This didn't seem any worse than the others so we kept Shae-Lynne on Carnation Good Start for a while.

After a few small weight gains Shae-Lynne was officially discharged from the hospital. However, we were to check in with our family doctor, Dr. David Pang, every couple of days for a weigh in.

Dr. Andrews wrote in the official discharge summary to Dr. Pang, in part, "Nurses corroborate mother that the baby is difficult to feed and it requires a lot of time, patience and skill.... We did some investigation toward metabolic problems and some reports are still pending (amino acids and organic acids) but all the others were normal.... I still have some concerns as it is abnormal that the baby does not feed well and requires fortified formula to grow."

The amino acids and organic acids report later came back as normal. Sounds, to me like they placed a small bandage over a wound they had yet to find. Shae-Lynne still had no diagnosis. We were still struggling with our hour-and-a-half long feedings. We were no better off.

I was still determined; Shae-Lynne was going to be breast-fed. Actually, I don't know if determined is the correct word—stupid and stubborn also come to mind. Still trying to produce enough, I continued to pump. I had kept this schedule for over one month and her weight gains were remaining mediocre.

* * *

As Dr. Pang continued to monitor Shae-Lynne at her daily weigh in, he witnessed poor weight gains and I continued to insist she wasn't eating and was definitely vomiting too much. He felt Shae-Lynne should be re-admitted and sent us off to see Dr. Andrews again.

The first thing Dr. Andrews did was to increase the amount of calories Shae-Lynne would be getting, from twenty-four to twenty-seven per ounce. At this point she was back to her birth weight, over a month old and finally back to seven pounds. Dr. Andrews also ordered a cranial ultrasound, a sweat test for cystic fibrosis (because of the amount of mucous that came up when she vomited) and, of course, the standard blood work and electrolytes. Again, everything came back normal.

After two consecutive weight gains (albeit small) Shae-Lynne was discharged once more and we continued our daily weigh in with Dr. Pang. This was Shae-Lynne's second time in the hospital. She was again being released with no diagnosis other than failure to thrive that we had heard after her first stay. Shae-Lynne was still vomiting about four to five times per day and would not eat. This time Dr. Andrews wrote in his letter to Dr. Pang, "I will see her again in two days for a weigh in, if we are still not doing well, I think we will have to bring her in for tube feeds until she fattens up a little bit more." This was the first time he spoke about tube feeding. He went on to say, "It is a little unclear as to why Shae-Lynne is not gaining all that well...." But it wasn't unclear. I had told the doctors over and over why—it's because she wasn't eating! I didn't need a medical degree to figure that out. The real question was *why* wasn't she eating.

Imagine that—all the tests, two lengthy hospital stays, three doctors and no one could tell Michael and me why Shae-Lynne would not eat and why she was vomiting so much. Our beautiful baby was about one month old and she had spent most of that time in the hospital.

More time passed. At two consecutive weigh in appointments, Shae-Lynne had lost weight so you can guess what came next.

Dr. Andrews admitted Shae-Lynne again. He said he just wanted to keep an eye on her and let the nurses see how she was eating and possibly have them feed her. Talk about reinforcing my fears about it being my fault. He might as well have said, "It's your fault." Of course, what he did keep saying was not to blame myself. Maybe he really didn't think it was my fault, but boy, it sure felt like I was to blame. I am her mother, if she is failing to thrive for no apparent medical reason, who else is to blame?

During this hospital stay, Shae-Lynne was prescribed a drug called Propulsid. The generic name is Cisapride. This has since been taken off the market, as it has been associated with abnormal heart rhythms in rare cases. Propulsid is what is known as a prokinetic, which speeds up the emptying time of the stomach. It also causes the lower esophageal sphincter (LES, lower part of the esophagus) to contract. This can help to reduce the amount of acid that may enter the esophagus. Propulsid is still available through special access programs in some areas. To qualify for these programs, an initial EKG and a follow up five days after the initiation of the drug will likely be done. Also there are risks for certain drug interactions. Propulsid is an adult medication.

For the first few days that Shae-Lynne was on Propulsid she did very well. She ate two ounces in record time without vomiting at almost every feed. Sadly, after about a week, Shae-Lynne was back to her usual vomiting. It was now decided to try Alimentum, a special hypo-allergenic formula designed for babies who have problems with other types of formula. Alimentum may be recommended to relieve colicky symptoms such as excessive crying and fussiness caused by sensitivity to whole or intact protein.

Shae-Lynne had a couple of small weight gains. She was discharged once more with no diagnosis. The daily weigh in and fighting to get her to eat began again. At one weigh in, Dr. Andrews brought up the subject of tube feeding. This would involve inserting a tube through Shae-Lynne's nose and down to her stomach. He thought she just needed to get a little stronger and then everything would be fine. He was sure she just didn't have the strength to eat due to not getting enough nutrition the past couple of months. I was assured that this was no big deal. They had plenty of kids being tube fed at home. They would give us a pump to take home and Shae-Lynne could be fed through the night.

This dramatically increased the pressure on me to get Shae-Lynne to eat and gain weight—I could not imagine anything worse than having all kinds of medical equipment in the house. I was picturing an IV stand beside her crib and it made me sick. Sure it was no big deal to Dr. Andrews, but it wasn't an option to me. Shae-Lynne would just have to get over this and I was sure she would. Although I must admit for a moment, the prospect of not having to be up all night trying to feed her was a bit appealing.

I decided to begin a dairy of Shae-Lynne's eating, sleeping and vomiting to help solve the mystery. I started keeping the daily intake, vomits, and reactions to what she ate. Below is a section of my journal. On this particular day, we kind of got off schedule but I didn't worry about it. I just desperately wanted her to eat.

Shae-Lynne was exactly two months old at this time without a diagnosis.

July 16, 2000
 3:30-5:00 a.m.—For about 45 minutes fought to keep her awake (after undressing her, etc.) Finally she came around a little

and screamed until I finally gave up. Once I stopped she settled down and went to sleep.

Total taken: nursed one side plus 40 mls (less than 1.5 ozs) Alimentum

6:30-7:15 a.m.—woke crying, gagged and choked, trying to vomit about five times but nothing came up. Couldn't get one drop into her, forced the bottle into her mouth, applied pressure, etc., just wouldn't suck or swallow at all! Eventually she went to sleep.
Total taken: 0 mls

9:00-9:20 a.m.—nursed one side and then went to sleep, I'm not fighting with her this time...will wait to see it she gets hungry approx. total taken: 15-30 mls (½ to 1 oz)

9:45-11:15 a.m.—woke crying—hungry? Still had to force her to eat, she threw up and I finally gave up
Total taken: 40 mls. (less than 1.5 oz)

11:30-12:00 p.m.—seemed hungry, I tried again. Took 10 mls then fell asleep, unable to wake her.
Total taken: 10 mls. (less than ½ oz)

12:40-1:15 p.m.—seemed hungry again but still wouldn't eat, screamed when I would try to give it to her and then threw up
Total taken: 15 mls (less than ½ oz)

1:20-2:15 p.m.—fought with intermittent screaming and sleeping and eventually gave up
Total taken: 50 mls (less than 2 ozs)

4:00-5:10 p.m.—wouldn't nurse for some reason, took the first 20 mls okay, threw up when I was finished
Total taken: 45 mls (1.5 ozs)

5:30-6:30 p.m.—slept on and off, very drowsy, best feed in a while
Total taken: 55 mls (less than 2 ozs)

7:00 p.m.—seemed hungry again so I tried again since her daily intake is so low. Took 20 well then went to sleep. I didn't push it
Total taken: 20 mls (less than 1 oz)

9:00-9:45 p.m.—excellent feed, a little pokey but not asleep
Total taken: 60 mls (2 ozs)

10:00 p.m.—she just threw up so I tried giving her more, nursed and she took 25 mls more
Total taken: nursed plus 25 mls (less than 1 oz)

DAILY TOTAL: 335 mls formula plus nursing (generous estimate: 100 mls)

VOMITS: 4 (estimate 120 mls [4 ozs])

I don't know what took longer—these feedings or the note taking. I kept this up daily for months.

Every time we saw Dr. Andrews and I explained how long it was taking to feed Shae-Lynne and the small amount she was taking, he would tell me to limit her feedings to one-half an hour. That's it, no more. Stop after one-half hour. He said I had to let her get hungry. Every time he suggested it, I told him no. I knew her better and she does not get hungry—if I limited her feeding time she would certainly lose weight. After he had made this suggestion a number of times, I decided to do as he had asked. Maybe if I listened to him and he saw that I knew what I was talking about, he would take matters more seriously. I stopped trying to force Shae-Lynne for two days and let her take what she wanted in a half hour. After that she received nothing until her next feeding. It was horrible, at least for me, she was never happier. She took no more than a half ounce (15 mls) in any one feeding and she would usually throw that up. After two days she stopped peeing and I couldn't follow this suggestion any longer. We went back to struggling with one and one-half hour feedings. I hated it, but I had to continue. The half-hour feedings definitely did not work. Dr. Andrews stopped suggesting it when he saw the results.

* * *

It was feeding time, three a.m. I crawled back into bed only an hour ago from the last feeding. I was beyond exhaustion and as I stood up I wondered to myself how I managed to stand. I was so tired. I dragged myself to Shae-Lynne's cradle, feeling as though I could cry. I picked her up and held her, trying to wake her gently (no one likes to be rushed when being awaked). Her little eyes opened, then closed for a moment. She opened her eyes again and looked into mine. As she looked into my eyes she reached up and touched my cheek with a slight grin. My heart melted and I sat on the bed with her in my arms as we shared this special time together. It was moments like these that I am most grateful for. It was so easy to forget everything else and just get lost staring at that perfect little face. This was why I was able to stand and tend to her needs. I had to. Shae-Lynne was more than worth it.

The feeding problems had been going on for two months, and I was losing patience with Shae-Lynne's doctors. I brought her to them to fix her and they still hadn't. Why couldn't they give me any answers?

One day her neonatologist, whom I didn't particularly like, told me for the hundredth time that I was stressed and needed to relax. "I could give you something to help you relax, you know," he said. I looked at him in disbelief. What was he talking about?

"What do you mean, medication?"

"Yes."

I laughed. I had to laugh at him, because if I didn't I surely would have choked him. He had to be joking knowing how much I was trying to make the nursing work. I'm sure he would've liked it if I had said, "Sure, drug me." Maybe that would shut me up, and maybe I wouldn't expect so much from him. I'd like to see this guy give birth, let alone experience what we had gone through in the last two months and not be stressed.

What reaction did he expect me to have if not stress after the events of the past few months? Shouldn't he be more concerned if I wasn't stressed? I know Shae-Lynne's doctors were only trying to help, but what they didn't realize was they were increasing my stress. The pressure of the daily weigh in alone was extremely difficult on me and they just wouldn't listen to what I was saying. How can they arrive at a proper diagnosis when they don't listen to the person who spends the most time with the patient?

CHAPTER THREE

MAYBE THE ANSWER

As time passed, I noticed Shae-Lynne was more alert for her feedings but she was starting to fight against accepting the bottle by screaming. She was arching her back and actually flinging her whole body backwards trying to get away from my offerings of food. It was hard to hold onto her. Her strength surprised me. Screaming became routine during her feedings. When I stopped trying to feed her she would settle down. Occasionally she would cry in such a way that led me to believe that she was hungry. That never meant she would eat any more or any better.

We went for another of our many appointments with Dr. Andrews and I described the new symptoms and change in her behavior. I felt this was the first time he actually heard my complaints about Shae-Lynne's excessive vomiting.

"I really think she has some reflux happening," he said.

"What do you mean reflux, like acid reflux—heartburn?" I asked. I don't mind telling you I thought he was nuts. I found it hard to believe, that everything we'd been through was because of heartburn. That's what pregnant women and old men who eat and drink too much will get. This was my misguided view of reflux.

"For sure, tons of babies have some degree of reflux when they're first born. There is a muscle at the top of the stomach that opens to allow food to pass and then closes to keep the food down. It's very common in newborns for this muscle to be underdeveloped and weak. This may cause a lot of spit up. Often acid from the stomach comes up with the food and burns. Many babies learn that eating hurts and this may cause them to not want to eat."

I liked and respected Dr. Andrews and felt he was a very good pediatrician; however, I was quite skeptical. "Okay, but Shae-Lynne wouldn't eat from the start. How do you explain that? And I've seen babies spit up, Shae-Lynne's not like that at all. What about the choking?" I questioned.

"Well, that, I can't answer. She has been a mystery from the beginning, that's for sure. We're going to send her for an upper GI to check for reflux. We will put her on Zantac for now to help reduce the acid pain." He headed for the phone to call radiology to see if they could squeeze her in then.

He hung up the phone. "Okay, you can take Shae-Lynne down now and they will do the upper GI. Come back here when you have finished the test." Conveniently Dr. Andrews' office was in the hospital so it was only a matter of heading downstairs for the test. "Don't worry, this test is quite easy and not at all invasive. They'll put Shae-Lynne on an x-ray table and have her drink a small amount of radioactive solution called barium. They'll watch a series of fluoroscopy x-rays of the liquid going down to her stomach."

"Simple? Are you kidding? How am I going to get her to drink the stuff?" I smiled a little jokingly. However, the question was a valid one.

"So what happens if it shows reflux? What will that mean?" Michael asked as we got up and headed for the door.

"Nothing to be worried about. There are several effective and safe medications available and she will outgrow it in a few months. Usually at about six months. When kids start sitting up on their own they begin to improve and then by nine months or a year, they outgrow it completely." He walked us out of the office. "I'll see you back here when you're finished in x-ray."

Michael and I felt hopeful as we walked down the long sterile white corridor toward the x-ray department for Shae-Lynne's upper GI. It sounded as if reflux was easy to treat and Shae-Lynne would outgrow it. *Whew, what more could we ask for?* We thought we were finally getting answers and more importantly, solutions.

Surprisingly, Shae-Lynne drank the barium with no problems. I was hoping it contained a lot of calories. She needed them. Okay, the test was over. Let's hear the results, please. Negative for reflux! Everything was normal. We were quite happy the test revealed there was no reflux; however, we were also very frustrated as we were back to square one—not knowing the cause of Shae-Lynne's problems.

We walked back up to Dr. Andrews' office feeling lost and frustrated all over again.

"So, how'd it go?" he asked.

"Well, Shae-Lynne actually drank the barium, but the test showed no reflux." I sighed.

"That's okay, upper GI's don't always reveal reflux. I just thought we'd give it a try. I still think that's what's going on here. I'm going to give you a prescription for Zantac. Even if it's not reflux the Zantac will help with the acid pain from the vomiting." Zantac is what is known as an acid blocker or Histamine H-2 receptor antagonist. These types of drugs are used to suppress the amount of acid in the stomach so that what is being refluxed and/or vomited is not so acidic and will not irritate or inflame the esophagus.

"How long before it starts to work?" Michael asked.

"Give it a week or so."

I left his office with mixed emotions. I was hopeful that Zantac was going to solve our problems but I was also very doubtful after all this that the solution would be this easy. Besides, I still didn't understand why the test came back negative for reflux and yet Dr. Andrews still believed it to be reflux. Some months later, I learned that although an upper GI is the most commonly ordered study and typically the first one administered, it is not the most reliable in diagnosing reflux. An upper GI is actually better for detecting anatomical problems, finding hiatal hernia and esophageal dysmotility (poor movement of food through the esophagus and into the stomach).

* * *

The weeks went by with no improvement and Shae-Lynne's weight gains were still very poor. There was no choice now, other than the insertion of the NG tube (N: Naso, meaning in through the nose and G: Gastric, into the stomach). She was to be admitted to the hospital yet again for a few days. The tube would be inserted for twenty-four hours while she was monitored.

Over the first twenty-four hours her vomiting continued and Shae-Lynne had not gained weight. It was decided to leave the NG tube in for several weeks, maybe even a month. All of a sudden I was being taught what to do with the tube and how to use the pump. I hated having to learn this stuff. I was a mother, not a nurse! It was also very important now for Shae-Lynne not to lie flat while her feed was running. If she were to lie flat, she could aspirate (food and stomach contents backup into the airway and lungs) and of course, throw up. This meant we had to put pillows under Shae-Lynne's changing pad, crib mattress and anywhere she was going to be lying down. At first it was very difficult to change her diaper while she was propped up so much. Eventually though, like everything else, we got used to it.

When we left the hospital, Shae-Lynne was on twelve-hour continuous feeds through the night. During the day I was to try to bottle feed her, at which time she was to get three ounces (90 mls) per feeding. Whatever she didn't take by mouth (with a time limit of half an hour), I would have to pump into her in bolus (larger amounts given over smaller periods of time) feeds.

Shae-Lynne would only take about an ounce or two (30-60 mls) by bottle. I would then have to get her formula and feeding pump ready and pump the rest into her so that she would get the necessary three ounces (90 mls). This had to be done consistently or she would not get the amount of calories needed to gain weight. It was around this time Dr. Andrews asked me to stop nursing and to express my milk. By giving it to her in a bottle he would know the exact amount she was taking. This was forcing me to accept that she was not going to be a breast-fed baby and I was not ready to give up—there's that stubborn streak again. Unfortunately, it was apparent the day the tube was placed down her little nose and throat as a means to feed her that I had to seriously readjust my expectations.

Perhaps it was so difficult for me to let go of the nursing because it was re-enforcing Shae-Lynne's special needs. To accept the tube feeding in place of breast-feeding meant accepting that my daughter wasn't "perfect." I was desperately trying to accept the reality of not having the fantasy child that I had envisioned, and I was holding in an incredible amount of guilt over not producing enough breast milk. She always did so much better on breast milk than she did on formula and so a part of me blamed myself for everything that was happening. If only I wasn't such a failure she would be fine. I think that realistically I knew that our problems were bigger than that. Maybe that's why I held on to so much guilt. If it *was* my fault and all she really needed was breast milk then maybe there wasn't anything wrong with her after all.

The only thing I knew for sure was that she almost never gagged or threw up when she got breast milk so she was going to get as much of that as I could possibly muster. I continued to express.

I was pushing myself beyond the limits of what I ever thought a person could handle. I can't even count the number of phone calls my mother received only to hear a crying and somewhat hysterical me on the other end. She is always so comforting, so positive, and always able to lift my spirits and get me through another day. Although I must say, a few quiet moments with Shae-Lynne along with her precious smile also seems to do the trick.

I was so happy when Mom came for another visit. Mom usually came once a year; now that Shae-Lynne was here this was her second visit and a third one was planned for December. Guess we know whom she wanted to see, but who could blame her.

My mom's plane arrived the day Shae-Lynne was to be released from the hospital. I picked Mom up at the nearby airport and headed back to the hospital for Shae-Lynne. Michael and I were getting used to seeing the tube in her nose. Although Mom always tried to be positive, I could see the tears in her eyes when she first saw Shae-Lynne at the hospital. Shae-Lynne seemed so tiny, so sweet and seeing her hooked up to this big monstrosity was hard on Mom. Shae-Lynne looked at my mother with fear. The hospital stay, tests, doctors, and tubes were beginning to frighten her.

Together we packed up everything: tubes, formula, toys, diaper bag, feeding bags, syringes. It took a few trips to the car but we were finally ready to head home. Michael was very anxious to see Shae-Lynne as he had not seen her since the previous day.

Now that Mom was here, I was sure together we would find the cure and fix Shae-Lynne but we didn't know where to look. Keep in mind Shae-Lynne was nearly three months old and we still didn't have a definite diagnosis. Mom and I starting searching online and at the library for anything we thought would give us some answers. Trying to come up with something, we felt like we were searching for a needle in a haystack. We gathered information on infants that vomit, failure to thrive, food aversions, reflux, and everything else we thought might be of help. All the articles we found reverted back to "call your doctor" if the vomiting persists. We were seeing doctors almost daily but they had no answers. Where do we go now? We were beginning to lose hope. Three months is a long time to watch your baby suffer.

During my mom's visit we had taken Shae-Lynne to the local hospital for one of her many NG tube replacements (she had pulled it out and I was certainly not going to be the one to re-insert it). Dr. Tardanico happened to be on call that evening. He is the same doctor who had referred Shae-Lynne to Dr. Andrews almost three months earlier when she was first admitted to the NICU. Dr. Tardanico had not seen Shae-Lynne since then and he asked me how she was doing. I warned him not to get me started and when he insisted that I tell him what had been going on, I broke down and cried.

I told him Shae-Lynne refused to eat, hence the NG tube. In spite of everything that was being done for her, she was still throwing up. She had not gained sufficient weight despite fortified formula and the NG. I further explained to him that although the doctor suspected reflux, we still had no real diagnosis. I asked how all this could be caused by reflux. He seemed angry that her symptoms had gone on for so long, and thought it was time for another opinion. He immediately made arrangements to get Shae-Lynne admitted to Children's Hospital, which is a four-hour ride away from our home.

Again I was a mess. Although it was nice to be validated and a part of me was anxious to find out what was really wrong, I was quite scared. It was settled though—we were going to Halifax.

We had a nice visit with Mom. One day we even pretended we were a normal family and took Shae-Lynne down to the lake. This was actually her first time out, other than going to the doctor's office or hospital. We took pictures and laughed. It was a nice afternoon, a two-hour getaway; however, it left Shae-Lynne late for a feeding. It actually took longer than two hours to get ready to go out. We had to mix formula, clean the feeding bags, bathe and dress Shae-Lynne, clean up vomit and change Shae-Lynne again.

Mom rushed me. She shouted at me, "Don't wash your hair. We have no time for that." We were on a very tight schedule if we wanted to go out.

Okay, I was all showered and Mom had Shae-Lynne ready to go for the second time. "Let's go." I had just barely finished speaking, when she puked on me again.

Mom said, "Never mind, let's go now!"

Yes, I had a wonderful afternoon walking around the boardwalk with dirty hair and puke on my shirt.

Now back to reality. Michael, Shae-Lynne and I headed for Halifax. Actually I was convinced that this was the answer, so much so that I didn't think we'd be coming back with the NG tube. I was naive enough to think they would be able to fix everything easily. Mom left for home. She was anxious to get there. She had a plan to help (although I was not to find out about that until later).

* * *

Michael took time away from work so that he could travel with Shae-Lynne and me. The four-hour drive seemed like eight. We finally arrived at Children's Hospital. Shae-Lynne's room was extremely large and the hospital provided us with two cots on which to sleep. Thankfully, we were both allowed to stay in the room with Shae-Lynne.

Once at Children's more tests were performed. Shae-Lynne saw a geneticist, a cardiologist (just to triple check her heart murmur), a gastroenterologist, two nutritionists, residents, students, and I can't even remember whom else.

The gastroenterologist, Dr. Robert Clements, ordered another Upper GI series, a reflux scan and a chest x-ray. He also felt it was reflux after discussing Shae-Lynne's file with Dr. Andrews. Dr. Clements, a tall middle-aged man, never seemed to have enough time to talk to us. Shae-Lynne had been admitted for three days before he even came to our room.

The chest x-ray showed that Shae-Lynne had been aspirating either food or refluxed material and we were concerned that she would have permanent damage to her lungs. We were assured that her lungs would filter out the aspirated materials and it would not likely cause any damage.

The reflux scan is very similar to the Upper GI. Shae-Lynne was given barium and then (after she threw it up three times) she was laid flat on a table that had an x-ray under it. The x-ray continually took pictures for one hour in order to measure the amount of reflux, if any. The scan showed significant reflux, even after she threw up most of the barium.

Reflux happens when stomach contents move up out of the stomach and into the esophagus. Everyone, regardless of age, has experienced this at some time. It's more commonly referred to as heartburn, although heartburn is only a symptom. The stomach has a lining to protect it from the hydrochloric acid produced to digest food. However, the esophagus does not. When acid backs up into the esophagus, it can cause a burning sensation. If it continues, damage will occur to the esophagus.

Reflux itself is considered a somewhat benign condition that does not require treatment. It does not lead to long-term complications, nor cause inflammation or affect growth and development. This is what is typically seen in infants. The majority of infants may outgrow this by the time they are twelve months old, or sooner. This is what I was led to believe we were dealing with. Later, I would do my own research and discover that there are different degrees of reflux. By sharp contrast, GER is referred to as Gastro Esophageal Reflux Disease (GERD) when it is accompanied by complications that require medical intervention. Shae-Lynne's complications (to date) have included severe food and oral aversions, poor growth, failure to thrive, esophagitis, aspiration, and both developmental and speech delays. Others include wheezing, apnea, anemia, pneumonia, Barrett's esophagus and apparent life-threatening events.

* * *

The doctors decided to do an endoscopy to show the extent of the damage done by the reflux. This is when a flexible tube (endoscope) with lights and a camera is passed down through the child's mouth into the esophagus, stomach, and duodenum (first part of the small bowel). The doctor is then able to look directly at the esophagus, stomach and duodenum to see if there may be any irritation or inflammation present. They are also able to take biopsies to check for any damage done from the reflux. Repeated exposure to the esophagus from stomach acid causes inflammation and damage to the lining of the esophagus called esophagitis. Biopsies will confirm if esophagitis is present.

The doctors explained that the test would be administered in the operating room (OR) and that Shae-Lynne would have to be sedated for the scope. They would need to insert an IV in order to keep her hydrated, as she would not be allowed food for a few hours before the test. After the test she would be taken to recovery and we could see her after she woke up.

When it came time for the test, Michael carried Shae-Lynne as we headed down to the OR. We were both so afraid for her, having no idea how she would respond to the anesthesia. After she was prepped, Michael gave her a kiss and passed her to me for a big hug and kiss. The nurse arrived. She took Shae-Lynne from me and carried her down the long white corridor. Michael and I took a seat in two rocking chairs and we waited. On the wall directly across from us was a large framed picture of a hundred different types of butterflies indicating the names of each. As I sat staring at all the different colored wings, I was becoming ill thinking about Shae-Lynne being held down while her little arm was poked over and over trying to insert the IV. I was jolted out of my daydream state when I suddenly heard Shae-Lynne scream all the way down the hall from the OR. I cried long after her screaming had stopped.

The test was to be approximately twenty minutes long. We thought that Shae-Lynne would be in surgery for about forty-five minutes including time to place the IV and for the medication to take affect. Over an hour and a half had passed before the nurse, at long last, came to us and said that Shae-Lynne was in the recovery area. There was no explanation as to why it took so long. She did say everything went well. We headed to recovery to wait until we could see Shae-Lynne.

After what seemed to be an eternity, we were allowed in the recovery room to be with her. Shae-Lynne was starting to wake up. We walked in the door, washed our hands and looked around the room for Shae-Lynne. It was a large room with many beds. One whole wall was painted with a mural of Snow White and the Seven Dwarfs and the ceiling had toys and decorations hanging from it. My eyes scanned the room for Shae-Lynne until I spotted her. As we made our way over to her, I was fighting back the tears. She looked so tiny, so frail, lying in a big bed with the sides pulled up. She had an IV in one arm and there was a small band-aid-like thing taped to her toe that was attached to an oxygen monitor. Her little face was red and even slightly swollen. Her eyelids were most definitely very swollen and she was so limp and still. I wanted to hold her so badly. The nurse told me to sit in the chair and she would pass Shae-Lynne to me. Picking her up was not a one-person job with all the wires and cords attached to her. Shae-Lynne stirred a bit and tried to cry when the nurse started to lift her. Her lips were so dry and parched that they were stuck together. She could barely open her mouth. It took several tries before she was able to make any sound at all. Her voice was almost non-existent, breaking up as she cried, almost like a bad case of laryngitis. Poor Shae-Lynne was so hoarse, the more she tried to cry the more upset she became. It was obvious that it hurt to make any noise. I cuddled and rocked her the entire time we were in recovery.

* * *

So there it was, Shae-Lynne had reflux. How could that be all that was wrong? I argued. I couldn't believe heartburn had caused all this. I begged Dr. Clements to give me the name of one person (or give my name to them for privacy reasons) who had gone through this much agony over reflux. I thought it was ridiculous when someone saw the tube in Shae-Lynne's nose and asked what was wrong for me to respond, "reflux." You should have seen the looks I got. Please, over and over I begged, I want to know one other person who had to tube feed their otherwise perfectly normal baby because of heartburn. I was always told that they see a lot of kids with reflux this severe but nothing more specific. I think this is an area in medicine that is drastically underrated. People tend to be drawn to other people that are going through similar circumstances. It's human nature to need to know that someone understands and has been there. I think doctors underestimate the value found in support groups and such organizations. It would've helped so much if they had pointed me in the direction of another family dealing with the same issues.

The biopsies collected from Shae-Lynne's endoscopy revealed she did, in fact, have esophagitis. Shae-Lynne's throat and duodenum were also inflamed. The inflammation in her throat was likely due to her vomiting and constant acid exposure, even though she had been on Zantac, an acid blocker. The inflammation in her duodenum was attributed to a milk protein allergy even though she was already on a hypo allergenic formula. "No more breast milk or milk products of any kind," they said; even though I insisted she did better on breast milk than anything else.

It is difficult to deal with daily living when you have a sick infant; however, it is more so when the medical profession on which you are relying simply will not listen to what you are saying. After all, I am her mother. I am with Shae-Lynne twenty-four hours a day. I see every reaction she has, good or bad, to everything that goes into her. I knew she was happy on breast milk. Goodness knows though, I had to do as I was told, far be it for me to go against doctor's orders. It was then that I finally gave up expressing and Shae-Lynne stopped getting breast milk. It took four months and doctors' orders for me to accept that the nursing wasn't going to work.

The tests also determined Shae-Lynne had delayed gastric emptying (DGE) which means that food doesn't empty into the intestines as fast as it should. This would leave her feeling full longer. Obviously if she feels full she won't want to eat. I have since read about fifty percent of babies with reflux also have DGE.

Since the doctor felt that Shae-Lynne also had a milk protein allergy, her formula was changed once again. She was now on Vivonex T.E.N. (Total Enteral Nutrition). This is an adult formula that is amino acid based. It is more elemental than its counterpart Vivonex Pediatric. According to the doctors, it is impossible to be allergic to this formula and that is why Shae-Lynne was put on it. Because it is an adult formula, I was given a recipe to modify the product for her.

Shae-Lynne was kept on Zantac and to that Maxeran (Metoclopramide) also known as Reglan in the US and Losec (Omeprazole) also known as Prilosec in the US were added. Maxeran is a prokinetic, which increases gastric emptying time; it causes the stomach to empty faster and increases the strength of the LES. Losec is a proton pump inhibitor. Proton pump refers to the site in the stomach cell where hydrochloric acid is produced and pumped into the stomach. It works by slowing or preventing the production of acid in the stomach. Because of the expense of proton pumps inhibitors H-2 blockers like Zantac are usually tried first.

During this hospital stay, Shae-Lynne's feeding schedule was changed. She went to nineteen hours on the feeding tube and off for five. I would attempt to give her a bottle after three of the five hours she was off. She would receive all the nutrition she needed during the nineteen hours on, so it really would not matter if she didn't take anything by mouth.

After two weeks, and a barrage of tests, we were sent home. We had seen no improvement from either the new formula or the new medications. The doctors were convinced that we would see an improvement in a few days so off we went waiting for her to get better. With this hospital stay, as with all the others, we left feeling as though nothing had been accomplished. We felt as though they didn't know what else to do so they would simply release Shae-Lynne, send her home and forget about her…as though they had fixed her.

The biggest change in Shae-Lynne after her two-week stay at Children's Hospital was in her personality. She now had an immense fear of people. If anyone other than Michael or I went near her she screamed. I realize all infants go through a strange stage. This was definitely different. It was heart wrenching to watch the change that took place in her.

* * *

It was now September. Shae-Lynne was four months old and weighed only 4.03 kilograms (9 lbs). Despite our best efforts, she was still considered failure to thrive and still vomiting. One night was exceptionally bad. Shae-Lynne always gagged and choked quite profusely. She had even stopped breathing a few times when she threw up, but this time she just kept choking.

Minutes passed and although she had stopped vomiting, she continued to scream, choke and cough. It seemed as though there was something caught in her throat. Yes, she was definitely choking on something. But what? I tilted Shae-Lynne's head back and tried to look inside her mouth, when all of a sudden she coughed again and I saw something yellow sticking out of her mouth. Her NG tube? It was the same color as her tube. How could it be? I could see the tube still in the proper place in her nose. As she continued to choke, more of the tube came out. I knew I had to do something. I was terrified for her and didn't really know what was happening. I loosened the tape that was holding the tube to her face and starting pulling it out of her nose. She screamed louder and choked harder. Oddly, for a moment, the more I pulled on the tube the further out her mouth it stuck. I had no idea if I was doing the right thing but knew I had to get the tube out of her mouth. With all the instructions I received from her nurses on how to deal with the NG tube on a daily basis (checking its placement in her belly, etc.), no one ever told me she could throw it up. I was not prepared for this. I kept pulling and Shae-Lynne kept screaming and choking. Finally the tube was out. She gave one last cough and she slowly calmed down as I sat rocking her. Eventually the crying subsided. When Shae-Lynne stopped crying completely, I laid her down and I was shaking. She looked up at me and gave me a big smile. I collapsed on the floor in a heap of tears. Another hysterical phone call to Mom.

So this is reflux. I was learning quickly.

* * *

Michael and I never expected anything like this. I thought back to the beginning when we saw "that little blue line." What happened to all our wonderful plans? We spent most of the summer in the hospital. I don't even remember what the weather was like, never mind picnics by the water. It is difficult to take your child out when she is hooked to a tube. Shae-Lynne's formula was in a bag hanging from an intravenous stand, attached to a heavy pump similar to an IV pump. You could not just pick her up and walk away. We also had to push a huge stand and carry her at the same time. It was really quite awkward. Every day was spent giving medicine, bottle feeding, tube feeding, cleaning bottles, cleaning and disinfecting feeding bags, keeping notes, cleaning vomit. Cleaning vomit. Cleaning vomit. Well, you get the idea.

When Shae-Lynne's schedule was first changed I was thrilled. Wow, five hours off, I thought, and no pressure to feed every three hours. When we got home and settled into our routine, I realized the new schedule was no improvement. Shae-Lynne was still vomiting often, which meant it was best to try to keep her still and not move her around. She could not lie flat while the feed was running, nor for about an hour after her feed was shut off (or she may aspirate and would surely puke). This meant that her bath and playtime were restricted to four hours. However, during the four hours I had to give her a bottle, which meant a half hour of feeding time (this was the limit) and another hour of motionless time. In reality I had about two and one-half hours a day to bathe her and give her floor/play time. Not much time left for any sort of life. This did not leave much time to learn and develop gross motor skills.

Below is another sample from my food/vomit dairy.

Sept 16. 2000
5:00 a.m.—threw up about an ounce
8:00 a.m.—threw up close to an ounce
10:00 a.m.—threw up close to an ounce
12:00 p.m.—shut off her feed 584 mls 24 hour total
12:40 p.m.—threw up almost an ounce
3:00 p.m.—nippled just over an ounce
5:00 p.m.—started feed again
6:30 p.m.—threw up an ounce
8:30 p.m.—threw up an ounce
8:45 p.m.—threw up again about a half ounce
Daily Total: 642 mls
Vomits: 7

Shae-Lynne's vomiting was slowing increasing. One day we hit a record of five. A week or so later we hit another record of seven in one day. At this time, Shae-Lynne's rate per hour (the amount being pumped into her over the span of one hour) was about one ounce. You will note that she was vomiting about an ounce per hour, thus canceling out an entire hour's worth of feeding time.

It was becoming increasingly difficult to handle this situation. I struggled to keep up my energy and focus all my attention on helping Shae-Lynne but watching her like this was insufferable. I was desperately trying to survive one puke or screaming fit at a time. Michael continued to work and he tried to help as much as possible. Bathing Shae-Lynne was his favorite time, she was always happy then.

Although Michael was extremely supportive, this was causing many difficult moments between us. We both knew that we had to survive this for Shae-Lynne's sake. She needed us both.

I knew our daughter's illness was just as wearing on Michael as it was for me. However, I didn't care. He didn't have to watch Shae-Lynne's pain every day, all day. Since our trip to Children's Hospital, she wouldn't stay with anyone except me (she even went through a short period of not going to Michael). I wasn't getting any breaks, none, ever. I couldn't discuss my feelings of disappointment with Michael. As with all men, he wanted to fix everything and got angry and frustrated when he couldn't. That didn't help me. I needed Mom so much because she was my sounding board. She was someone to complain to, someone to cry to. Unfortunately, I was beginning to feel guilty every time I called her to cry. I am sure it was just as hard for her. Maybe even harder, as she couldn't be with us to help as much as she would have liked. She didn't realize just how much listening helped.

CHAPTER FOUR

YOU ARE NOT ALONE

While we were in Halifax, Mom was putting *her plan* into action, which was still unknown to me. Mom wanted to help so she went to her local newspaper office to ask for assistance. They kindly obliged by running the following story. Of course, this was done before the official word that it was reflux we were dealing with.

Our story in part, "a plea for help":

Shae-Lynne was born on May 16th. She is nearly four months old and does not want to eat. She is being tube fed (through the nose) for nineteen hours a day. The other five hours she is bottle fed (will not take more than an ounce). She vomits much of what is fed to her; sometimes uncontrollably to the point where she is unable to breathe and also chokes. On one occasion she vomited so forcefully that the feeding tube was pushed out of her mouth.

She has been in the hospital most of the last four months. Although much testing has been done—her medical problems remain a mystery to the doctors. They have been unable to help. Today she remains in a local hospital and will be sent to Children's Hospital (four hours from her home) once again.

If anyone has experienced anything similar to what is happening to Shae-Lynne—please write, e-mail, or call with your comments and suggestions.

My mom also contacted several doctors-turned-authors whose books she had read. She prayed that they were caring enough to respond. Maybe they had answers that would help us.

The calls started coming in. It was such an incredible and wonderful feeling for Mom, knowing there were so many people reaching out to help. After speaking with these people, my mother later told me, "You could hear the excitement in their voices. They felt sure they had the answers. They knew their information would help Shae-Lynne."

Calls came in from nurses, feeding specialists from well-known hospitals, occupational therapists, etc. People called who had children (or knew of children) who were being tube fed. This was not new to them.

Of course, had I known what my mother was up to I would have been quite angry, and certainly wouldn't have understood why she went to newspapers or what she was trying to accomplish. I must say though, once she finally did tell me what she had done and gave me the names of the people who contacted her, it was the first time that I didn't feel so completely alone. After I got over the anger I was glad for what she had done. What a great learning experience this was and definitely uplifting that these people really cared. Yet, it was also sad because some of the calls Mom received were from parents or friends of seriously ill infants. These infants were tube fed because of mental retardation, Down's syndrome, or cerebral palsy, etc. They were living their own problems and still took the time to contact Shae-Lynne's Grammy Jean.

I'll never forget Mom's excitement the day she called to let me know that she had received a handwritten letter from Dr. Bernard Siegel—better known as "Bernie" (author of *Love, Medicine & Miracles* and *Peace, Love and Healing*, among others). It was difficult for her to put into words how touched she was. She told me that when she read his books she felt as though she knew him; she could feel his love and sincerity. Bernie began to e-mail me and sent along a massage kit to help Shae-Lynne. I thought that was such a loving and caring thing to do. He explained how infant massage could aid in infant growth, as well as digestion, not to mention the closeness it brought to mother and baby.

It seemed that the readers of the newspaper article were also searching for answers. When you're desperate for an answer, almost anything sounds logical. One caller suggested goat's milk. Mom thought, "Yes, I think that would work." Several thought it sounded like pyloric stenosis (the muscle at the bottom of the stomach is too thick or blocked); however, that had been ruled out. Many felt if we demanded a certain test be performed, we'd find the answer. Another caller suggested a chiropractor; perhaps a problem occurred during delivery to put something out of place. Mom thought, "Yes, that may work." Medications that may help were suggested. Could it be "celiac disease"? (Faulty absorption of food in the intestines and characterized by diarrhea and malnutrition).

Many people were convinced that if we would bring Shae-Lynne to *their* doctor, he/she could help. I think it is wonderful when one has such great faith in their doctor. Over and over Mom heard, "Bring the baby to Children's Hospital in Boston. They will find out what is wrong."

Mom heard many stories about young children and kept hope. However, she wanted to hear from or about someone who had "outgrown" reflux, as she had heard so often is the case. Each day, Mom was anxious to check the mail and messages. It was exciting for her to receive a handwritten note from Dr. Mona Lisa Schulz (author of *Awakening Intuition*) noting she had passed Mom's inquiry to her friend Dr. Christiane Northrup (author of *Women's Bodies, Women's Wisdom*, among others). Dr. Northrup, in turn, was to pass the request along to her mother. You see, some forty years ago, Mrs. Edna Northrup had dealt with a similar experience. It was wonderful and very much appreciated that Mrs. Northrup called Mom to share her story in detail. Tube feeding was definitely more difficult back then.

Along with calls, Mom was also receiving cards and letters. She kept notes, phone numbers, and e-mail addresses for future reference. Mom felt it was now time to let me in on what she had done so that I could deal directly with the responses. I was ready to speak or e-mail firsthand with the people whose family members were experiencing the same medical problems. I made many friends and they continue to this day. At first Mom hesitated to tell us what she had been up to. She was afraid I would be angry, since she was bringing our personal business out in the open. I knew she did it out of love because she wanted to help. Shae-Lynne's problems were not going to disappear. It was encouraging to know that we did not suffer alone.

I filled Mom in on the information we received from the hospital, the official diagnosis—reflux. Now it was time for her to contact the newspaper again with an update and thank all who had responded previously. Mom received more calls, more letters and more cards. This time she passed them on to me directly. We were now receiving answers specifically about reflux. More friendships began.

The responses we received from the second newspaper article opened many doors. Our greatest support came from others who were experiencing what we were. Greta was my first ray of hope. She had responded to mom's "plea for help." Greta lives in Texas and was visiting her mother in the Boston area when she read the article. Mom told me, "God works in funny ways." As usual, I thought she was being a little dramatic but I did have to admit it a bit odd that Greta happened to be in the same town as Mom at the same time the article appeared.

Finally someone understood. I was not crazy. I was not overreacting. I did not need to be medicated. I was a normal mother, hurting because my child hurt. I was hurting because I was unable to help Shae-Lynne. Greta and I communicated regularly via e-mail and later exchanged photos by mail. She had been and was still addressing on a daily basis the same issues I had been trying to get others to understand. Following is part of the e-mail I received from Greta.

Scott's Story (as told by Greta, his mom)

Scott was born full term, normal weight. He is my second child (both boys). I nursed Daniel, my first son, for fourteen months, and introduced solid foods around seven months. I noticed when Scott was almost four months old he was not gaining weight. I complained to my pediatrician that he was not nursing as I felt he should be; however, she told me I was overly concerned. At his six-month visit, he was delayed and his weight according to the charts was below normal. I switched pediatricians; Scott was hospitalized that day for malnutrition/FTT. I was breast-feeding exclusively (my supply seemed to be down, as he was such a poor eater). Many lactation consultants tried to get my supply up. I continued to breast-feed for two more months. A weigh in before and after nursing indicated he was only taking in one to two ounces of breast milk. An NG tube was inserted and kept in for six months. Scott caught up developmentally within two weeks.

There were a lot of hospitalizations and tests. The tests included: MRI, ERG, EMG, barium swallow, GI series, Endoscopy (scopes), pH studies, lots of blood and developmental tests, RAST tests (allergy), ENT exam down his nose.

The doctors we have seen are: Developmental pediatrician (my main organizer; you need a good ringleader), pediatric nutritionist who deals with feedings, OT, PT, speech pathologist, developmental psychologist, behavioral psychologist, neurologist, endocrinologist, pediatric GI, geneticist, lactation consultant, ENT, social worker, home health nurse, allergist, and dentist.

We kept thinking he would outgrow it, so we didn't want to do a gastronomy (surgery to insert feeding tube into the stomach). Unfortunately, Scott pulled his NG tube out so often (sometimes I replaced it six times a day); his nose would swell so bad we had to us Afrin to get it back down. At one year, a Ph probe revealed he had severe reflux. A fundoplication and gastronomy were done right away. Scott was a silent refluxer, as he NEVER threw up. He had a Nissen procedure. For the next two months we experienced many complications as the button sight never healed properly. Scott is now 2 ½ years old. He is normal developmentally.

Scott never wanted food until he had his fundo. Some days he eats and others he does not—very unpredictable. We have gone as long as six weeks without supplementing to see if he would pick up eating on his own; he lost three pounds the last time (which he can't afford to lose). The doctors continue to run tests and we still get other opinions. We are just hoping he grows out of it!

I feel like I have so much to tell you. I have made some mistakes with his care. It can put a lot of stress in your marriage and within your family. My parents are still mad I won't take Scott to Boston Children's Hospital. We have grown stronger as a family and are very close. We enjoy every second with both our kids. Our oldest one definitely had a lot of tough times, while Mom was gone.

Greta and I became friends and continue to be. I loved having someone to talk to who understands reflux.

* * *

Next, Claudia got in touch with me about her daughter Hannah. As she told me her daughter's story, I could not believe how similar feeding time was between our two babies.

Hannah's story (as told by Claudia, her mom)

I had a wonderful normal full-term pregnancy and easy delivery with Hannah. She would not eat since the day she was born. Immediately after birth, I struggled to get her to eat. Nursing first, then with the bottle. We thought it would pass. Hannah was less and less interested in feeding. She never cried for food or exhibited any signs of hunger. For me, it was becoming very stressful right from the beginning. She is our second baby, so I had a sense that this was not the way it was supposed to be!

Hannah lost more interest in feeding. She seemed very uncomfortable after eating. Developmentally, she was very normal in every other way. The feeding difficulties continued. I told the doctors Hannah seemed to have an aversion to eating. (Which I think they quickly disregarded.) I had been force-feeding her. She quickly began to associate the bottle/feeding with unhappiness. She would cry uncontrollably. I attempted to feed her; she would turn away and adamantly refuse to eat. It was as if it was causing her pain. If I did get some into her, she would get so upset at times that she would gag and spit up. She never woke at night to feed, and if she did she would take a couple of sips, swallow, then squirm around as if it hurt her tummy and stop eating.

At ten weeks of age, she completely stopped eating. Hannah was admitted to Children's Hospital in Boston, they were concerned about dehydration. In the hospital, she was given an IV and we were supposed to see a feeding specialist (as she had refused to eat for nine weeks). Hannah also had an upper GI/swallow study performed; that was rough. She refused to drink so they had to inject the Barium through a tube in her nose. They were able to rule out a malrotation and any other anatomical abnormalities. They said she might have reflux and a milk allergy. They wanted to start her on Zantac and changed her formula to Nutramigen. It had not specifically shown up on the upper GI but they said that it doesn't always—the baby would have to be refluxing at THAT moment in order for it to be conclusive. However, the feeding specialist would not see us because they thought they wouldn't have an accurate consult because Hannah was congested. I was pretty much devastated.

According to the doctors, it was not critical, as Hannah was stable, not actually losing weight. The fact of the matter was that the child did not WANT to eat—she did not desire/cry for food or show ANY signs of hunger. I tried everything to get Hannah to eat. I always felt as if we were one feeding away from a feeding tube. I also knew how much caloric intake she should be taking in a day and was struggling. We were stranded to our house and feeding schedule.

After the hospital stay we also consulted with Early Intervention here in Mass. They offer physical therapy, speech therapy, occupational therapy, etc., all free of charge. They have come to our house, her day care and still see her one to two times a month. They gauged her development—physical and cognitive—and have tracked her this whole time. They told me that Hannah presented herself as if she was a preemie—weak suck, distracted eater—apparently they see feeding difficulties quite often with preemies. I didn't think too much of it at the time, because Hannah was not premature, but that ended up being the source for where I ultimately found people who experienced what I had and information! They also told me that it did not look as if it was neurological. Usually they can see other signs such as un-parallel movements on one side of the body vs. the other, etc. I thought things would get better when we started solids because I could spoon feed her and maybe she just didn't like the bottle. That didn't work.

At seven months old, things accelerated. Hannah had her monthly weight check, was seeing the nutritionist for a weight check two weeks later and getting dietary suggestions and seeing the GI two weeks after that. The GI examined Hannah and said she looked "great"—try to increase caloric intake to get her weight up (yeah, right, I almost said, you try to feed her more). He took a stool sample and ordered blood work. He wanted to test for food allergies, malabsorption, etc. He also ordered a sweat test for CF, just precautionary. After reviewing the tests Hannah was switched from Nutramigen to Neocate for protein intolerance. ($40 a can lasting less than a week). We were also preparing it so it would equate to 27cal/oz as compared to 20 in regular formula.

Watching her food intake, I'd just get five ounces into her, and she would burp, gag, and the whole thing would come back up. She was spitting up anywhere from one time per day to five or six (after each bottle). Hannah seemed to have a hyperactive gag reflux and had trouble with more solid textures. It was devastating. I was still trying to do everything on my own— the doctors didn't have a solution. Things got worse as she approached nine months and I thought she was going to have to go on a feeding tube. The doctors had said reflux and milk allergy was the problem, but that did not explain the failure to eat. Nothing had really helped so far. It was as if her brain was not triggering a response of hunger and want for food because she never even wanted food after eleven hours (most babies want to eat after two to four hours). She hadn't even woken in the middle of the night when she was a newborn for bottles like most all babies do in the first weeks.

On the Internet, I learned of an antihistamine, Periactin (generic name cyproheptadine), known to be an appetite stimulant. Sometimes it's given to babies that won't eat and for other people with illnesses that lead to loss of appetite (anorexics, etc). I was so thrilled at the possibility that something might help. It was a last straw because a feeding tube was not far away. After much insistence, the doctor allowed us to try it. It has been a BIG difference, a lifesaver. Hannah now eats and sometimes even asks for food.

Although we STILL haven't figured out exactly what's going on, Hannah is a thriving, very happy, lovable eighteen-month-old. It's hard but we do everything we can to get her to eat. Without the Periactin, she has absolutely NO appetite. We weaned her off it a couple of months ago and it was very difficult. She completely reverted back to not wanting to eat and every spoonful was a fight. Now we're getting by day by day!

This has truly consumed our lives the past eighteen months—I am always worried whether she is getting enough and it has been at times physically exhausting. I know that I struggled and felt very alone because I was not getting any answers and couldn't find much if anything about this problem.

It was good to hear that Hannah appears to be improving and hopefully recovery is near.

* * *

Shortly after I met Greta and Claudia I stumbled across a support group for parents of reflux children. These parents had joined the group to share their stories and offer support and helpful suggestions. Eventually I found a whole reflux community of moms who have come together to comfort each other through this difficult disease and I have since found over a half dozen more support groups for parents of reflux children. I also found support groups for moms whose children are tube fed and I was amazed at how many of them were tube fed because of reflux.

I began reading some of their children's stories and each day I would log on to read the daily posts.

- *My son is three months old; he is gaining weight so the doctors don't think his case is severe. They do not see the crying in pain. He was on Zantac, Pepcid, Mylanta, nothing helps. I do not even mind the throwing up. I just want his pain to stop.*
- *I wish someone could offer a solution besides "he'll outgrow it"; that means nothing when you see real tears streaming down the face of your screaming baby.*
- *Reflux is a nightmare. My oldest is suffering from lack of attention. My daughter is now on Zantac. I got Prevacid today, but am afraid to try it. She couldn't take Reglan, Bethanocol or Donperidone—they all made her hyper and irritated.*
- *My ten-month-old grandson had a G-tube put in ten days ago and has had increased vomiting since then. The surgeon did tell my daughter that G-tube placement could make reflux worse. Has anyone had this experience?*
- *My seven-month-old daughter stopped eating a few months ago. Has been on Zantac, Reglan and Losec. Nothing helps. She still vomits and REFUSES to eat. Most of her nutrition is through the NG tube. Help! Any suggestions?*

It is hard for me to express what I felt when I began reading these stories. At first I felt excited because there is such a sense of camaraderie and so much emotional support. Then, I was shocked. I began to realize the horrors of reflux and my eyes were opened to the seriousness of this disease. Babies everywhere are suffering. Their parents are devastated and struggling daily for some peace and reassurance.

I think what shocked me the most was that Shae-Lynne's reflux could have been worse. We could have been dealing with getting no sleep from her being awake all night screaming. We could have been dealing with apnea monitors and wondering whether she would stop breathing in her sleep. I never realized that I was lucky that Shae-Lynne only did that when she was awake and throwing up. We could have been dealing with frequent and reoccurring aspiration pneumonias, asthma, anemia, etc.

I was relieved to find people who understood. These people would not automatically judge me. They would not think that I was doing something wrong because my child would not eat. These parents understood how unmanageable it is to do five loads of laundry a day. They know what it is like to make an appointment and always be late because you are cleaning up vomit and changing both your clothes and your baby's clothes several times before you go out the door—only to have her throw up again in the car. Can you imagine doing all this while carrying your new little bundle of joy in one arm and the feeding bag, pump (about the size of an intravenous pump) and diaper bag in the other? Oops, I forgot that extra formula in a cooler also must go along. That's not even to mention the aggravation of the tube itself—either it's too long and getting stepped on or caught in something, or not long enough and pulling tight on her nose and face. These people understood. Wow, it was nice, and a lot of them had been dealing with this stuff for years and had a lot of good suggestions. I made many new friends and they were truly my life line for months.

The more I read, the angrier I became. These women, as with myself, had turned to their children's team of doctors over and over again looking for help. They were usually dismissed as overreacting or they would hear as I had, "Wait for your child to outgrow it." In desperation some turned to the so-called anti-reflux surgery, feeling it was their final option, only to have their children still miserable with the same problems or with new problems caused by the surgery.

I want the general public to know the seriousness of this condition. I want everyone to know how few alternatives there are. How can research be done without money and how can money be raised without awareness? It is of no consequence to me that a large percentage of babies born with reflux have no complications and may outgrow it. Everyone seems to know this. But shouldn't the minority that don't outgrow it and live in constant pain be the ones that get attention? Why are doctors still performing the same surgery for reflux as they did over forty years ago? Why don't more people know how devastating this disease is?

In some cases the complications from GERD can be fatal as Ms Shimberg, *Coping with Chronic Heartburn*, learned first hand when her uncle Marty Weill died of Aden carcinoma of the esophagus. He died nine months after having been diagnosed.

I have a mission: to raise awareness. I believe that everything happens for a reason, I had to believe that to survive. I don't know why Shae-Lynne was born with this disease but I had to try to make some good come of it. Could Shae-Lynne have been born with GERD so that I could try to help others? Probably not, but I couldn't help her and I was so tired of feeling useless that I had to try to help someone. I wanted to give these little refluxers a voice and give their moms hope, as I had found.

My mother with her many attempts to help, along with my anger over reading of how many children were suffering, really got me moving. I was inspired. I contacted every television station I could think of, some local, some not, and told them of what these kids are going through. I was sure it was compelling enough to get them to do the same research I had done and put together a very informative story.

Mom was also doing the same thing in her area, with much disappointment. There are medical advisors on these stations, yet they show no interest as, "It's only reflux, they grow out of it." She told me how angry she was as she watched the news: a thirty-second clip on whales, a thirty-second clip about a woman who sells lemonade on the corner, and a thirty-second report of the death of someone involved in an accident. Mom contacted the station again and posed the following questions: "If Shae-Lynne dies next week from choking on her vomit—will you be so kind as to report that? Will reflux be important enough then?" She finally received a call back and heard the same disappointing response, "Your granddaughter is not from this area, and there is no interest here." This story was not "about her granddaughter"; it was intended to be about infants all over the world experiencing and suffering from this disease. Why won't they listen? We know the answer. It is because, "It's only reflux, they will outgrow it." If only they would listen, they would understand the severity of this condition.

With attitudes like the people mentioned above, no one would ever know how serious reflux is.

Until GERD is a household word like asthma or diabetes there will be no chance of finding a cure. I think of the people calling to raise money for these diseases and so many others, but who is collecting for GERD? Doesn't this seem serious enough for some extensive research? For goodness sakes, reflux is now being said to actually *cause* asthma in some cases. The two very definitely go hand in hand. If this were more understood I think the asthma societies would be interested in studying the correlation.

At least I did have one welcomed response. Our local station contacted me and wanted to do our story. When writing to the television stations, it was my hope that they would do some research, present facts and make more people aware of GERD. The station agreed to do the story if I went on the air and told Shae-Lynne's story. It took me a few days to think it over, as I definitely did not want to appear on television. I knew I had to do it though. I knew there were other people going through this trauma and if they felt as alone as I had when Shae-Lynne's illness began, I knew they needed to hear our story. It aired the following week.

I thought I could make a difference. I did not feel that I was helping Shae-Lynne, but perhaps I could offer comfort to other desperate parents who thought they were alone. People were now calling me and asking for information, help and suggestions. A short time before this I was the one desperately searching for answers. Now I was helping others not to feel so alone.

One woman called, "My seven-month-old boy is up all night, every night crying. What can I do to help him?" I felt so badly for her because I knew there was nothing to be done. She had his crib elevated and he was on Zantac. I told her of Losec and Maxeran and suggested that she ask her pediatrician about them. She told me how glad she was that I had done the story and thanked me for the information.

Another mother called to say that her child had been experiencing difficulties similar to those of Shae-Lynne. However, her doctors had no idea that it could be reflux. She was so grateful that I had done the story and that made it all worthwhile. Her child's pediatrician immediately scheduled the upper GI. Now they had something to go on.

My next project was a website. I designed a site with Shae-Lynne's story and reflux information. I truly welcome reading and sharing stories with all these reflux moms and learning first hand of their experiences.

CHAPTER FIVE

REALITIES OF REFLUX

I knew a lot more about Shae-Lynne's condition now, and I had many new friends going through this, too. Why did I not feel any better? Shae-Lynne was getting worse. She was eating less and throwing up more. We hit another record—ten vomits (six to seven was average at this point) in one day.

We were off to see Dr. Andrews for another checkup and weigh in. At five months old Shae-Lynne weighed 4.75 kgs (10 lbs). Dr. Andrews decided to admit her again because of the increase in vomiting. I had also told him she stopped breathing when she threw up. Not much was done for Shae-Lynne at the hospital—a couple more tests and blood work. Dr. Andrews consulted with Dr. Clements, Shae-Lynne's GI at Children's Hospital, to chart a new plan of action.

* * *

Dr. Clements said the next step was to change Shae-Lynne's NG tube to an NJ tube. N for naso, meaning through the nose and J for jejunum meaning positioned through the stomach and duodenum (first part of the small bowel) into the jejunum (second part of the small bowel). This would mean her food would be pumped directly into her small intestine and there would never be anything in her stomach to be refluxed. The upside of the NJ tube was if she did vomit, it should only be gastric contents. Thus, Shae-Lynne should begin to gain weight. The downside to the NJ tube was that she would have to be on twenty-four-hour continuous feeds. Unlike the stomach, the bowel is not able to handle large quantities of food at one time. The other downside to the NJ is that if it had to be replaced, Shae-Lynne would need to go to the hospital again to have it inserted under fluoroscopic x-ray to assure proper placement. Obviously, this would make it extremely inconvenient if and when it needed to be replaced. We were discharged to await the placement of the NJ tube.

Shae-Lynne's doctors and actually anyone who thought they understood what reflux is had originally told us her reflux would probably start to improve when she was about six months old. Now that we were getting close to that six-month mark, they were starting to extend the time frame, now saying at nine to ten months we would begin to see improvement. Increasing her feeds to twenty-four hours a day was going to completely eliminate any hope of her ever having any kind of appetite. Slowly Shae-Lynne was drifting further and further away from eating on her own. I was losing what little faith I had left.

* * *

Shae-Lynne began to stop breathing much more frequently when she was throwing up. It was happening at least once a day and was terrifying. I had visions of us rushing her to the hospital to be revived. This child was going to drown on her own vomit. About a week and a half before our NJ appointment, I called Dr. Andrews to find out what I could do to help Shae-Lynne when she stopped breathing. So far I had been lucky and she would start again on her own; but I feared for the time that she wouldn't be able to get her breath by herself. He told me there would be nothing I could do and that Shae-Lynne would require medical attention if she didn't start breathing on her own. He was extremely concerned and decided to admit her to our local hospital for a week and half, as a precautionary measure, while we waited for the NJ placement.

* * *

Shae-Lynne's first Halloween was spent driving to her next hospital appointment, which was at Children's Hospital at nine a.m. the following morning. Since the hospital was four hours away, we had to head up the night before. The morning they were to insert the NJ tube, I had to shut her feed off at six a.m., as she had to have an empty stomach for the procedure.

When we arrived at the hospital the radiologist informed us that the procedure could take some time. It is difficult to get the tube around the curves of the duodenum (first part of the small bowel) and into the jejunum. For fifteen minutes Michael and a nurse had to hold Shae-Lynne down (I stood in the corner in tears) while she screamed at the top of her lungs and threw up continuously. My heart ached. Poor Shae-Lynne, she cried so hard she made herself sick over and over again. We were told everything went well as often times it takes longer and we were really glad when it was over.

I was not allowed to start Shae-Lynne's feeds until we saw Dr. Clements, which was to be at two thirty that same day. I had no idea what to set her rate at now that she had the NJ tube. That meant Shae-Lynne went almost all day without food. That was the last thing she needed when she wasn't gaining weight. Not that she minded, no food to Shae-Lynne meant a great day. Not once did she get hungry and once the trauma of the tube placement was over she didn't have any pukes all day.

We wandered around the hospital most of the day waiting to see Dr. Clements. Finally at almost four p.m. (he was running late) we saw him. He gave me the rate at which he thought we should start Shae-Lynne's feed, weighed her and measured her height. Dr. Clements said that the insertion of the NJ tube would probably cut her vomiting down to about half of what it was. He sent us home, not even knowing how she would respond to this method of feeding. I had no idea what to expect and I don't mind telling you I was a little irritated.

* * *

A couple of hours into the drive home the battery went dead on the pump. *Great*, I thought. *Shae-Lynne hasn't had food all day and now she has to wait another two hours until we get home.* I was extremely concerned about getting calories into her and also didn't want her to become dehydrated. I decided to use a syringe and manually give her formula. Unfortunately, not being prepared to administer her food in this manner, I only had a one ml syringe handy. It was almost seven p.m. so it was dark outside. I was in the back seat of the car beside Shae-Lynne. Michael was driving. I had the one ml syringe, an open container of formula and the end of Shae-Lynne's NJ tube and I was going to feed her. I was unable to see anything and I was trying to push one ml at a time into her tube. What a mess. By the time I found the opening of the tube to insert the syringe, we'd hit a bump and I'd lose it. It was very important that I kept track of how much she was getting so I had to count each one I had given her. Being afraid I'd lose track I asked Michael to repeat my counting. One, one...two, two...three, three...thirty-five, thirty-five...and so on. We continued this way for the next two hours until we arrived home.

As we journeyed closer to home, I was covered in formula and I began to laugh out loud. I was thinking about my friend who had a baby around the same time Shae-Lynne was born. She had probably just finished giving him supper; certainly not the way Shae-Lynne was getting hers. I had to laugh at myself feeding Shae-Lynne with my one ml syringe. I had to laugh or I would have cried. I don't think anyone can imagine or believe what I had to do just to get food into my beautiful little Shae-Lynne. Even I couldn't believe it.

"What are you laughing at?" Michael asked.

"Can you believe what we go through to feed this kid?" I must have been over tired to be so giggly because it certainly wasn't funny.

The first few days after we arrived home, we didn't see much improvement in Shae-Lynne's vomiting. She even started a new schedule of screaming inconsolably every night around six for about two hours the first couple weeks. For those two hours I would prop her on my shoulder and walk around the house trying to distract her. I played music, rocked her and sang to her. There was nothing more I could do but wait for the episode to pass. I suspect that moms of colicky babies could relate to this. Although with colic there does not seem to be a reason for the screaming, conversely, it is excruciating when you know your child is in pain.

Eventually, the evening screaming stopped and we finally saw improvement in Shae-Lynne's vomiting. She had cut down to about three to four per day. We could even lay her flat on the floor, which we were unable to do before. Things seemed to be going well. Unfortunately, by now Shae-Lynne wouldn't take any food by mouth. I knew she was slowly becoming more dependent on the tube feeds, but there was no need to worry about that now. Michael and I felt some relief as her vomiting had decreased and we would take what we could get. It strikes me odd how relative everything is— a few months ago three or four was an average day and now it was like heaven.

Mom missed Shae-Lynne and came for her third visit. Because Shae-Lynne was so terrified of people, I was afraid she would not let Mom near her. They bonded the minute they saw each other at the airport. She went right into my mother's arms. Mom didn't leave her side the entire visit. I remember that one day, Mom and Shae-Lynne were stretched out on the rug reading books together. Shae-Lynne reached over and grabbed Mom's face. I got a picture at just the right moment. It actually brought tears to my eyes, happy tears, to see her and Mom so close.

Although it was a short visit, I was so thrilled to see Mom. I think Shae-

Lynne was glad too because for the four days that my mom visited, Shae-Lynne only threw up one time. This was truly a miracle—only once in four days. Mom had received many phone calls, and listened to all the horrors: the puking, the times Shae-Lynne stopped breathing, and the crying in pain. Now that Mom was here, Shae-Lynne was really doing great. It was the best she had done since, well, since the beginning.

We had a nice visit and then Mom was gone again.

About two weeks after my mother left Shae-Lynne starting having bad days again. It started slowly and before I knew it, she was right back up to her ten or more vomits a day.

I called Dr. Andrews again. He decided to bring Shae-Lynne in to have the tube placement checked. "Maybe it's moved up into her stomach," he said. We went for yet another x-ray. "It looks perfect, exactly where it should be. She must just have a stomach bug."

I knew it wasn't a stomach bug. It had gone on too long for that to be the case. But why was she puking so much again? How could she be throwing up so much with no food in her stomach? The doctors were no help. They were unable to answer these questions. This was agonizing. I was so sick of desperately turning to her doctors for help and getting nowhere.

The next couple of weeks the excessive vomiting continued and Shae-Lynne began to scream and throw up throughout the night. All along the only thing we had going for us was that she was a fairly good sleeper and really didn't throw up much during the night. I knew I had this to be grateful for, as I had read so many other women's stories about being awake all night and rocking their screaming infants. Now Michael and I were the ones up at night with the screaming infant.

It was getting harder to get through the days, as we were not getting enough sleep at night. Out of desperation I called Dr. Andrews, it was now Christmas time and, of course, everyone was on holidays. The answering machine said in case of emergency go to the emergency room. I knew there was no use in doing that so *we waited* until the holidays were over. Alone, we fought to cope.

* * *

It is six a.m. and I am awakened by the sound of Shae-Lynne gagging in her crib next to our bed. We keep her crib in our room, as it is easier to have her nearby when she wakes throwing up. With another gag she begins to cry.

I cringe and hope she will settle herself and fall back to sleep. This is the fifth time since I had put her to bed that she woke gagging. The other five times ended in Shae-Lynne puking. My eyes are so heavy and tired I don't even think I can open them. I pray she will go back to sleep. This is now the new routine, like clockwork every night. Michael and I are both worn out and we begin to take our exhaustion out on each other.

Shae-Lynne is screaming now. As I drag my weary body out of bed, I hear another gag that sounds wet. If I don't get to her in time, the front of her sleeper will be soaked—oh no, too late. She lets out another cough and my first instinct is to grab her out of the crib. I am not thinking clearly. As I grab her in an effort to keep her from vomiting on her clothes and try to calm her down, I forget that I don't have a towel handy. Just as I lay her on my shoulder, my hair, arm and shoulder get soaked. Michael came to the rescue with a towel and threw it on my shoulder to cover the mess she has just made so she doesn't lay her head in it.

Just as he places the towel down her little head plops onto my shoulder and she's asleep again. I sit for another minute making sure she's finished. Shae-Lynne had a habit of settling down and then throwing up again just when I would think she was done. Ten minutes pass, she must be done now. As I begin to get up from the bed, sure enough she starts again. UGH! This time she isn't even awake so I hold her head up while Michael cleans her face. Another few minutes of puking and she is done, I think. As I lay her back in the crib I remember that her sleeper is wet from the first puke that I missed. I give it a good wipe with the towel to dry it the best I can. It doesn't seem to bother her and I really don't want to wake her and risk making her sick again so I don't bother to change her clothes.

I remove my puke-covered nightgown, slip into a clean one and climb back into bed with puke in my hair. At this point I didn't even care. Of course, I knew what a horrible mother I was by putting Shae-Lynne back to bed with puke on her nightclothes. I lie awake feeling guilty. I notice the time and wonder if we had actually gotten any sleep at all.

* * *

The holidays were over and I called Dr. Andrews. "Please," I begged, "you have to do something to help Shae-Lynne. She's miserable and we're exhausted. *Please*. There has to be something you can do. What would you do if she were *your* child?" I cried and pleaded with him to listen. I was sure if

I could just make him understand how much she hurt that he would do something to help her. Realistically I knew there was nothing he could do.

Dr. Andrews told me to bring Shae-Lynne in to see him the next day and he would squeeze her in. He was always so good at seeing her at the last minute. When we arrived there he admitted that he really didn't know what to do with her. Dr. Andrews had told me several times over the past months that he had never really seen a baby like Shae-Lynne. He mentioned getting another CT scan, perhaps there was a neurological cause to her vomiting that had not been detected in the first scan. He also said he would call Dr. Clements for suggestions. We headed home to await a CT scan appointment and to hear from Dr. Clements.

I wanted so desperately for Dr. Andrews to fix everything. After I hung up from each call, I felt guilty. I knew I was expecting the impossible from him. The stress from living this nightmare was never ending. It seemed that when things became too unbearable, I'd call Mom or Dr. Andrews. I knew with each phone call I also brought them pain.

I worried myself sick over the possibility of a neurological problem. I knew from my research that reflux this severe is more common in children with neurological problems and I knew that Shae-Lynne's development was falling behind. I imagined all kinds of horrible diseases. What if she had something degenerative and was going to start losing her milestones only to eventually become severely handicapped? Or worse, what if it was fatal? This was torture. I couldn't think about it anymore or I wouldn't be able to function.

I received a call the following day from Dr. Andrews. It seemed that the next step, according to Dr. Clements, was to do the jejunostomy. I knew from my research that this was surgery to insert a tube into the side of Shae-Lynne's belly directly into her jejunum, thus, eliminating the NJ tube. I had read that it may be possible for nasogastric or nasojejunal feeding tubes to exacerbate reflux from the LES being held open all the time.

Dr. Clements thought that by removing the NJ tube and replacing it with the J-tube we would see some improvement. I was furious! He didn't have any idea what to do with her next so he wanted to cut her open in the *hope* that *maybe* it would help. I had long since lost faith in his suggestions, although up until now none of them had been excessively invasive. It is easier to agree to try something when it doesn't involve surgery. I admit to not being very rational at this point.

Based on everything I had read I knew that the feeding tube down Shae-

Lynne's nose could not stay long term. It can cause damage to the nasal cavities and sinuses if left in too long. Dr. Andrews had assured me from the beginning that Shae-Lynne's nasal tube was short term and I just knew that Shae-Lynne would be eating before she would need surgery to replace her tube. This was not something that we were supposed to have to consider.

* * *

Since the doctors didn't have any other suggestions, a surgery consult was set up so that Michael and I could meet with the surgeon to discuss Shae-Lynne's options. We had already decided that there was no way we would allow her to be cut open for any reason. I felt as if I was preparing for battle as I started researching again. I had to find some way to stop this. I would go to this appointment well armed with alternatives.

Mom and I still felt that a great deal of this reflux problem may be related to diet and/or some kind of allergy. Diet was a good place to start. Shae-Lynne had been getting worse on the Vivonex T.E.N., so it was time to try something else. I had read about some moms trying goat's milk with their infants and children. I had asked Shae-Lynne's dietician months earlier if we could give goat's milk a try. Her response, as I expected, was no. I now was desperate. We had to try something else or surgery was next. I knew Shae-Lynne always did well on breast milk (although the doctors had not listened to me), so I decided on my own to give the goat's milk a try. Please don't think I am endorsing going against the advice of medical professionals. I definitely am not. Always listen to your doctor. I just knew that I had to try something, as nothing the medical profession had done or prescribed to date had helped. After all, she certainly couldn't get any worse.

I researched the nutritional values of breast milk, formula and goat's milk so that I could compare them. I wanted to be sure Shae-Lynne would get the proper amount of much needed fats, proteins, etc. needed for growth. Goat's milk has much more protein than infant formula and must be diluted with distilled water. Because it is being diluted with water, it also must have a carbohydrate source added to increase its calories to the normal twenty cals/oz. For example, in twelve ounces of goat's milk you need to add sixteen ounces of distilled or purified water and one to two tablespoons of brown rice syrup (rice syrup may be substituted with two to three tablespoons of barley malt) for calories. Goat's milk is low in folic acid and vitamin D so that should be added also. I must stress *that you should not switch your infant to goat's milk as a substitute for formula without your doctor's close supervision.* This is only an example. Present it to your doctor or nutritionist before using it for your infant.

For twenty-four hours I switched Shae-Lynne from Vivonex T.E.N. to the modified goat's milk and she did much better. Her vomiting decreased almost immediately and the gagging and retching almost stopped, just as it always had while she was on breast milk. This just reinforced my thoughts that she was not tolerating her formula. It was very clear to me that the improvement was from the change in formula. Within twenty minutes of switching I had witnessed an enormous difference. I knew that I could not keep Shae-Lynne on goat's milk long term because she needed to get twenty-seven calories per ounce and the goat's milk only gave her the twenty cals/oz. She needed more calories to gain weight. I was unable to dilute the goat's milk enough to lower the protein and still keep her calorie intake high enough. After seeing the improvement with the goat's milk I switched her back to Vivonex, not knowing what else to do. After twenty-four hours of doing well on goat's milk, within twenty minutes back on the Vivonex, she was gagging and puking. It felt like I was poisoning her. The difference was like night and day. If I hadn't seen it myself I would not have believed it. Taking goats milk certainly didn't cure Shae-Lynne, but she was definitely better. I knew she couldn't stay on the Vivonex T.E.N. and the goat's milk wasn't a long-term option so, not knowing what else to do, I decided to switch back to Carnation Good Start. Shae-Lynne seemed to improve a bit. I was also noticing that she did well when she was initially put on a new formula but would get increasingly worse the longer she was on it.

In my research, I found an article on formula rotation in infants written by Suzanne Evans Morris, Ph.D. of the New Visions Feeding Center in Virginia. These same principles can be found in *Is This Your Child?*, a book on allergies written by Dr. Doris Rapp. It explained how the human body was specifically designed for a diversified diet. The principle is to use four completely different formulas over a period of four days, switching formulas every day. On the fifth day you would go back to the first formula and so on.

The "rotation diet" made sense to me so I decided to present this as a possible plan of action to Dr. Clements when we went for the surgery consult. I made sure I had enough information so that I could present four different formulas to use as well. I decided to present Compleat Pediatric (beef, fruits and vegetables), Good Start (milk and corn), and Neocate (amino-acid based). I realized that I was only presenting three formulas; however, I was very nervous about introducing a soy-based formula, remembering how Shae-Lynne threw up the Isomil so many months earlier. I also knew that if I switched her formula every day and she had a reaction to one it would be difficult to know which one. I decided to discuss with Dr. Clements and the dietician the possibility of trying a modified version of the rotation diet. My suggestion would be to use three formulas and switch every week. Until then, Shae-Lynne would remain on Good Start.

Another article by Dr. Morris explained that excess mucous production is a way for the body to eliminate something that is harmful. As Shae-Lynne always threw up excessive amounts of mucous, it appeared that perhaps the formula was exacerbating the problem. I truly believed that there was something that caused Shae-Lynne's reflux to be so severe. Perhaps I had stumbled onto a possibility.

Around this time, while waiting for the surgery consult, I had heard from a very good friend of a woman operating a nearby Holistic Health Service. Her patients were having excellent results. Michael and I agreed we would take Shae-Lynne to her. I made an appointment at the alternative healing center where they performed a type of allergy testing called BEST testing, followed by some acupressure treatments. I was often ridiculed for taking Shae-Lynne for treatments. Michael came with me whenever possible, although he too had his doubts. Mom was one of the few people who stood behind me in this. If there were the slightest possibility of Shae-Lynne being helped, then we would go for it.

Paula, a tall slender woman, looking much younger than her actual years, was a very pleasant and soft-spoken person. I liked her immediately and so did Shae-Lynne. She held Shae-Lynne in her arms and they worked so well together.

The first thing Paula did was to put Shae-Lynne on digestive enzymes. They had papaya leaf, marshmallow root, slippery elm bark, aloe-vera leaf, catalase, stomach intrinsic factor, lipase, amylase, cellulase, vitamin B-12 and folic acid.

As time passed and Shae-Lynne had been on the digestive enzymes for a while, I saw that she began to gain weight. Of course, I cannot prove that it was because of the enzymes. Unfortunately, our insurance did not cover the cost and eventually we were unable to continue the treatments. It was extremely disappointing to stop these sessions especially since it was the first improvement in Shae-Lynne that we had seen. It was suggested that if we had a referral note from Shae-Lynne's doctor that the insurance might cover the expense. However, Dr. Andrews would not help with this request and the letter that Dr. Pang wrote on our behalf was rejected. Maybe someday alternative treatments will be honored, as they should. I do not know if they helped or would have had we finished the series. However, I do believe the enzymes helped Shae-Lynne have a few good weight gains.

* * *

In the meantime, the CT scan was scheduled and completed. Dr. Andrews called us with the results. He was concerned, as there appeared to be extra fluid around Shae-Lynne's brain that was not seen in the first CT scan. He was going to arrange an appointment with one of the neurologists at Children's Hospital. I was sick. We had to wait and wonder, well, we had to wait anyway. I tried my best not to think about it.

* * *

Finally, we went for our surgery consult. We discussed the J-tube placement and even the possibility of a fundoplication. Later I read the surgeon's report to Dr. Clements and in it he said that he didn't think a fundo would benefit Shae-Lynne. I don't know whether or not that was good news. On one hand he was agreeing with me that it probably wouldn't help her. On the other hand, this was supposedly the final alternative—when all else fails kind of thing. Yet, here he was saying he didn't think it would help Shae-Lynne. Well, if that won't help her, *what will?*

Our next appointment for that day was with Dr. Clements and the dietician. I told them that I had changed formulas, and there was no way I would ever give her the Vivonex T.E.N. again. I told them I had started Shae-Lynne on Good Start and she was doing better. I further insisted that Shae-Lynne did not have a milk-protein intolerance that they had stated was one of her problems. They grudgingly agreed with me since Shae-Lynne had done so poorly on Vivonex.

Next, I brought up my plan of the rotation diet. Although they refused to acknowledge the possible benefits of a rotation diet I made it clear that I was going to try it with or without their help. I explained to them the formulas I wished to try and when I mentioned the Compleat Pediatric, the dietician suggested I try that before doing anything else. She had heard favorable reports about it. The dietician said she would look into getting the Compleat for Shae-Lynne to try. I was thankful for her help.

After many phone calls, it was ultimately discovered that Compleat Pediatric was not available in Canada. It would, therefore, have to be ordered by my mother, sent to her house and then she had to send it up to us. That is what we did the whole time she remained on Compleat. Nothing was ever easy with Shae-Lynne.

* * *

One day while I was bathing Shae-Lynne, she started to throw up and it was an unusual color. Usually it's just gastric juices and mucous that comes up (gross, I know, sorry) but this time it was an odd brown color. I was worried as I wondered what was going on now. It actually appeared to be the same color as her formula. *It can't be the formula,* I thought. *She doesn't have any formula in her stomach, as it goes straight to her bowel.* I was very concerned as she continued to vomit all formula. Then, in an instant the tube slid out of her nose, out from underneath the tape on her face and landed in the tub with a plop. I stood in shock for a second as the formula from the tube began to flow into the tub. I shut the pump off and was in tears. This is unbelievable. All I wanted to do was give the kid a bath. Now I had to clean out the tub, refill it, and re-bathe her, never mind that I also had to get her to the hospital to have the tube replaced. She was covered in puke and the tube was full of formula. Why did *everything* have to be such a challenge?

Eventually I got the mess cleaned up but I was confused and very uneasy. How could it have just fallen out like that? It was pushed way down into the second part of her small bowel. I pictured the screen that the radiologist watched when he was placing the tube. All the way down into her stomach, out through the bottom of her stomach, and in and around, twist and turn after another. Somehow it must have been slowly working its way up from her bowel until it finally just fell out with a few violent retches. I wondered for how long it had been dislodged. Had it moved up to say her airway and somehow been pumping the food into her lungs for a time? No, it couldn't have been doing that or she would have been coughing more. I hope.

The NJ tube could not be replaced at our local hospital. However, Dr. Pang did insert her NG tube again until we could see a radiologist. Michael and I feared that Shae-Lynne, now getting formula into her stomach, would be awake all night screaming and vomiting. After all, she was already doing so poorly.

To our relief, Shae-Lynne slept through the night and her vomiting actually seemed somewhat improved. As time went on, Shae-Lynne seemed to be doing okay, so we decided not to have the NJ redone. We would wait to see how well she did with the NG. *Waiting again.* And hoping. Was this improvement from the Compleat Pediatric and the acupressure treatments with Paula? Could it be that I had finally done something to help Shae-Lynne?

CHAPTER SIX

SHAE-LYNNE'S FIRST TRIP

While we waited and watched to see how Shae-Lynne was going to react to the NG tube we took a trip to visit my mom and Jay. It was our turn, as Mom had made so many trips to our home. Of course, with Shae-Lynne it was a little more difficult for us to take a trip. I did not get my hopes up and did not make definite plans, as we never knew what surprises Shae-Lynne would throw our way. It was terrifying to think about taking her so far from home while she was so sick. I just had to put that out of my mind and hope that everything went well. We definitely needed a break.

Up to this point, we were still using the intravenous style pump attached to the huge stand. After pricing the various portable pumps and discussing with other moms which style was the best to get, I decided on a Zevex Enteralite. This particular model is slightly bigger than a Walkman and it would run in any position. The only problem was the cost. Obviously with everything Shae-Lynne had been going through, I had not returned to work. Without that second income it was next to impossible to come up with the two thousand dollars it was going to cost. I called everywhere I could think of and finally found a government program that was set up to fund just this type of thing. It was just a matter of waiting for the new portable pump to arrive so that we could take our trip. I was very excited about the freedom that would come with this portable pump. It would fit in a small shoulder bag. I guess you could say Michael and I were beginning to accept that this was long term.

* * *

We left around bedtime on a Thursday night so that Shae-Lynne would sleep during the drive. Hopefully she would not get too restless from being in the car for such a long time, as she would sleep most of the way. After I spent over an hour packing all of Shae-Lynne's things (extra feeding bags, medications, battery charger for the pump, syringes, formula, extra tubes just in case, the old pump and extra bags for it just in case), and a short time packing our suitcase, we were on our way.

It took us about fourteen hours to drive to Mom's house. Shae-Lynne slept most of the way, with the exception of a few throw ups and a few whines. It was so nice to be on vacation, even if we were still dealing with all the same issues. We arrived at Mom's early Friday morning shortly after she had left for work. I called her when we arrived so she wouldn't worry; I know it was difficult for her to be at work with us at her house, she was anxious to Shae-Lynne. I was glad to have some quiet time to shower, unpack, and relax. Jay surprised us by taking the day off from work and coming to visit.

Mom had not seen Shae-Lynne since December when she was only seven months old. Shae-Lynne was now ten months old and beginning to take steps if you held onto her hand. When Mom arrived home from work she was greeted at the door by Shae-Lynne walking toward her. Actually, when we arrived we found a walker for Shae-Lynne all set and ready to go. Shae-Lynne did very well. She was so proud of herself. She did have difficulty making turns. However, the night before we were leaving we realized Grammy Jean had put it together backwards. Michael corrected the problem and now there was no stopping Shae-Lynne.

Mom had no crib available so we made due with a borrowed newborn bassinet. Shae-Lynne was ten months old, and still fit into a newborn bed. We took the cradle part off the swing and placed it on the floor. We had to place a few towels under the mattress to give it height so that Shae-Lynne would not be flat. We also rolled up extra towels and placed them on the sides. Shae-Lynne slept snug as a bug in a rug. She was so adorable, more pictures of course. And Mom was out buying more towels.

We shopped like crazy. Shae-Lynne was always very good in stores. It was such a novelty to her that she sat quietly in her stroller and stared at everything. One day we were in Osh Kosh shopping for Shae-Lynne and she got a little fussy. Mom and Michael decided to take her out of the stroller to allow her to stand on her own for a minute. Shae-Lynne, because of the walker, was feeling very grown up. I, of course, being the shopaholic that I am, was completely oblivious to what they were doing with her. I was off in my own little corner of the store, with my armload of goods. I was enjoying the fact that I was more than ten feet away from Shae-Lynne for the first time in almost a year.

Mom came running over to me shouting, "Quick, quick, we have to go, Shae-Lynne is throwing up."

"So," I said, "she's always puking. What's the big deal?" Apparently she was puking on the floor of the store and they couldn't find the towel we had brought. Michael had his hands full of throw up. Shae-Lynne's clothes were covered and it was now going all over the floor of the store. As usual she was screaming and tears were pouring down her face.

Michael was kneeling on the floor next to Shae-Lynne. He was angry to be covered in puke.

Mom was running around in a panic. "Shae-Lynne messed her diaper, too. We have to get her out of here and clean her up."

Amateurs, I thought, I'm used to this. "Okay, okay, Ma, just give me a minute to pay for these things. I'll be right with you."

"No, there is no time for that. Give them to me and I'll take care of it. I'll be along shortly."

I was a little irritated to be rushed out. It certainly wasn't the first time Shae-Lynne was covered in puke. Paper towels were found to clean up the mess. I didn't see what the big deal was. It worked out pretty good though, since Mom grabbed my armload of clothes and all the new outfits were on Grammy Jean.

It was a nice mall with rooms set up for moms to change their infants. However, Shae-Lynne is not a normal infant, although we do try to treat her as normal as possible. In the changing room we could not lay her flat because of her reflux. Michael was trying to stand her up and keep her still and I was trying to change her diaper and clothes. Mom, standing in the corner, started to laugh hysterically. This got us all a little giddy. I think she realized that maybe she had overreacted. Without the salespeople and customers staring at us we relaxed a little and could laugh about it. We had to learn to laugh at things like this, once Shae-Lynne would stop screaming.

We changed Shae-Lynne's clothes and decided to head for home. On the way back to the car we stopped once to put her hat back on (she didn't like wearing hats and took them off frequently) and where we stopped a towel was lying on the ground. We all burst into laughter again. It was the towel that we must have lost the first time we passed by that spot. We had a few more shopping trips before we went home but that was by far the most eventful.

Of course, we always had people commenting about the feeding tube. "What's wrong? Is she sick?" I always became so frustrated. *Of course, she's sick!* I felt like screaming, *don't be so stupid!* Did it ever occur to any of these people that maybe I just wanted to go shopping and was too exhausted to field their foolish questions as their healthy little bundles ran around their feet yelling that they were hungry?

* * *

One of the people who had contacted Mom after the newspaper articles were published was an occupational therapist, Lisa Iarossi, OTR/L. Lisa specializes in sensory integration disorders (SID) in children. She is licensed and registered in Massachusetts and does a one-on-one private service. She said that many children with SID have feeding difficulties and/or frequent episodes of vomiting because of over sensitivity to textures in their mouths. I had heard from some other reflux moms that their children developed SID from years of reflux pain. I contacted Lisa when we arrived at my mother's house in the hope that maybe she would see Shae-Lynne. Lisa was sure she could make a difference with Shae-Lynne and agreed to take time from her busy schedule to see us. We were only visiting for a short time, so we truly appreciated her altering her schedule. Michael and I were so excited. More hope, maybe this would help Shae-Lynne.

Mom, Shae-Lynne and I arrived at Lisa's about nine thirty a.m. after approximately a forty-minute drive. We pulled up to a big beautiful home set on a hill with a few toys scattered over the front yard. Lisa came to the door and I was surprised that she seemed to be so young, probably about my age. A thin, pretty woman with dark hair and a kind, caring nature that was obvious from the beginning. We felt very welcomed. I knew right away I liked her. Shae-Lynne was a bit shy and fussy that day. Lisa was very patient and did not push herself on Shae-Lynne. She has two young children of her own. Lisa was on the verge of laryngitis when we arrived. By the time we left nearly two hours later, she had no voice left at all. She had planned to spend about an hour working with Shae-Lynne but we were there much longer.

Lisa explained a bit about SID, in particular, oral motor sensitivity. Often if a child has a very sensitive gag reflex, an odor, any food (with or without texture) or a nipple touching the lips, tongue or cheeks could cause a child to gag and therefore vomit. She gave many helpful suggestions. Among them, an oral motor exercise—a NUK brush, which is used to decrease oral motor sensitivity so that kids don't gag as easily and won't vomit as much.

During our visit, we also discussed Shae-Lynne's overall development. Lisa encouraged me to pursue occupational, speech and physical therapy evaluations and treatments to not only address Shae-Lynne's oral motor sensitivity but also her speech and language skills, fine motor skills, gross motor skills and her overall ability to process sensory information.

We had a great morning, became friends and have continued to keep in touch. I only wish she were closer. Lisa has since sent me instructions to help Shae-Lynne with her gross motor skills that have become somewhat delayed.

What a great vacation we had. Shae-Lynne let her Grammy Jean, Grampy Greg, Uncle Jay and Auntie Karen hold her and play with her. I was so pleased that Shae-Lynne was so good in trusting my family. She had been through so much and it seems to take her some time to let anyone get close to her. However, here she was perfectly comfortable with these strangers. We took lots of pictures, seven rolls to be exact. Grampy Greg and Uncle Jay fell hopelessly in love with her. After all, how could they not? Shae-Lynne can be such a little charmer.

Michael and I noticed a big difference in Shae-Lynne. The trip had been good for her. She had so many new experiences. She had grown so timid with all the trips to the hospital. With this trip, Shae-Lynne was meeting new people and every one of them loved her. So many of Mom's family knew the problems we had been having. We heard the same comments over and over. "She is so cute." "She doesn't look sick." "She isn't that small." I remember one day in particular when we were having a nice visit with Auntie. (Auntie is actually Mom's aunt, and although miles separate us, I have always felt very close to her. I was anxious to visit her.) Auntie was so pleased to meet Shae-Lynne. It seemed as though she couldn't believe some of the horror stories she had previously heard about Shae-Lynne. Within minutes, Shae-Lynne started to vomit and choke. That told it all.

Before we knew it, it was time to go home. We packed up the car and after a nice supper and many tears we started the long drive home. Again we were lucky as Shae-Lynne slept almost the whole way home.

* * *

Now that we were home and back to reality, I knew we had to think more seriously about having Shae-Lynne's J-tube surgery. Logically I knew that even if it didn't help her to stop vomiting, she needed to have the nasal tube removed. Many moms told me that it would be easier to deal with and more comfortable for her. The thought of surgery was so hard to accept. Every time I thought about it I broke down into tears and every time Michael and I discussed it he became angry. Yes, it was definitely the hardest decision we have ever made. And yet, it had to be done, it was a no-win situation.

I had to convince Michael and in my heart I didn't want surgery anymore than he did. Then there was the problem of my weak stomach. I am one of those who get weak and sick to my stomach at any little thing. How would I manage to clean and maintain an opening in Shae-Lynne's stomach? I knew there was no way I could handle that. How would we ever make this decision?

I guess Shae-Lynne must have known how difficult this surgery decision was for us because she decided to give us no choice. Within a few weeks of coming home from Boston she started to throw up more than ever. To make matters worse she was throwing up her tube again. This time it was happening every few days. Within a two-week span we had to have her tube replaced about eight times. It was so incredibly traumatic for her each time. With each vomit episode (over ten a day) I never knew from one minute to the next if it was going to end peacefully or if it was going to end with another trip to the hospital.

I called Dr. Andrews and told him that we needed to have her NJ replaced as she was throwing up way too often and she was frequently throwing up her tube. He made an appointment for the next day to see the radiologist again. While we were at the hospital I remember explaining to the radiologist how she had often been throwing up her tube and I asked if she would be able to throw up the NJ tube. She assured me that Shae-Lynne could not and that I had no need to worry. She apparently didn't know Shae-Lynne, our little baby super puker!

I think our surgery decision was made for us the night that Shae-Lynne threw up the NJ tube. It was at bedtime around nine o'clock. We had just gotten her settled down. She was in her pajamas and I had her night feed running when all of sudden the gagging and throwing up started. Again, Shae-Lynne screamed and choked excessively. By this time I was used to the different ways that she choked on the tube so I knew it was caught in her throat and was coming up. Again I started pulling it out for her like I had done so many other times in the last couple of days.

We really didn't want to go into the hospital right then and we considered leaving the tube out until the next morning. I was worried that Shae-Lynne would become dehydrated and knew she wouldn't gain weight. After we thought about it for a while, Michael and I decided to leave it out until the morning. I would take her into the hospital first thing in the morning to have it replaced and try to give her a bottle through the night. We came to this decision for two reasons. One, we were curious to see if Shae-Lynne would eat anything. Would she get hungry and know what to do about it? And, two, we also really wanted to give her little nose and throat a break from the tube. She was always like a different kid when she didn't have the tube in her nose. She was just happier and more comfortable. We knew Shae-Lynne would sleep well this night.

Every couple hours through the night I got up and tried to give her a bottle. She screamed and pushed it away every time. First thing in the morning I tried the bottle again. Still Shae-Lynne screamed and pushed it away when I brought it to her mouth. She did the same thing with the little bit of cereal that I tried to give her. It was now nine o'clock a.m. and she had nothing to eat for twelve hours and had no interest whatsoever in taking anything. We headed to the hospital to have the tube replaced. Unfortunately, there was no doctor available until eleven a.m. This meant Shae-Lynne would have gone for a total of fourteen hours without nourishment. Just before the tube was replaced, I tried to give her the bottle one last time and she still refused to take it.

The surgery decision was now a little easier to make. It was clear that Shae-Lynne was not going to eat any time in the near future. With her vomiting up a tube that is pushed all the way down into the second part of her small bowel, we obviously had to do something. I called Dr. Andrews and told him to arrange an appointment for the surgery. Oh yes, and are you wondering about the neurologist we were supposed to see? I mentioned to Dr. Andrews that we had not heard about the appointment that was to be scheduled with the neuro. It was so horrible waiting, not knowing. I spent every day trying not to think about it, but it was always there, the uncertainty and dread looming in the background. I got off the phone with Dr. Andrews and cried.

CHAPTER SEVEN

THE SURGERY

Approximately one month had passed since I initially called Dr. Andrews to have him set up the surgery for Shae-Lynne to have the jejunostomy (surgery to insert the feeding tube in her belly). During this month I had actually called his office several times to remind them. This was the hardest thing I had ever done in my life. Why did they make it harder for me? Why didn't they just set this up immediately? Actually, it was probably a matter of them waiting for the OR, not that they weren't trying to schedule it. A nurse from Children's Hospital finally called to book the appointment. She gave me a date that was two months away as that was the first one available. I hung up the phone and cried. How could we go on like this for another two months? Just then the phone rang again.

It was the nurse from the surgeon's office calling back. "We do have an opening for Shae-Lynne in two and a half weeks. Would that be better?"

"Wow," I said, "that soon?" My heart sank. She must have heard the fear in my voice as she then told me that if I wanted to keep the first appointment it was fine. She just wanted to give me the option. "No," I stopped her, "this has to be done, please book the new appointment." I was then told that the nurse from pre-op would be calling within a day or two, as I would have to take Shae-Lynne in the day before for pre-operative testing. I hung up the phone sobbing.

Almost as much as I hate what this disease is doing to Shae-Lynne, I hate what it is doing to me. This crying, blubbering mess is not me. I'm better than that. I'm stronger than that. Or so I would have thought. *What is wrong with me? I have to pull it together.* I just can't believe how hard this is. Every day is such an effort to get through. Every time Shae-Lynne throws up I swear I can't take it anymore and I just want to scream. It's agonizing to watch someone you love more than life itself in so much pain. This endless struggle to cope was getting the best of me.

This was really happening. I had so many conflicting emotions. A part of me was looking forward to the surgery. I had hoped it would make life a little more comfortable for Shae-Lynne and I was certainly looking forward to seeing her beautiful face without a tube stuck to it with globs of tape. There was also a part of me that felt sick at the thought of it. Were we really making the right choice for Shae-Lynne? I could not stand the thought of them cutting her open and I was heartbroken that we had gotten to this point.

A few days after the appointment was made for Shae-Lynne's surgery I finally received a call from the neurologist. We had an appointment with him the week before Shae-Lynne's surgery. I was a bundle of nerves the entire four-hour drive to Children's Hospital. *What was he going to tell me?* Michael couldn't leave his job so one of my closest friends since high school, Bev, came along for the drive to keep me company. Luckily, chatting with her seemed to shorten the drive.

I was so relieved to get there; I thought I'd have an answer once and for all. You would think by now I would know better. Dr. Peters, Pediatric Neurologist, said based on the reports he had seen, he was almost certain that the excess fluid was not causing Shae-Lynne to vomit. He went on to say that he would like to see the CT scans himself to be certain. *What?* I thought. *I just drove four hours and have another four hours to drive home and you don't even have the CT scans here?* Apparently no one had the foresight to courier them to Dr. Peters. He asked that I get them from the other hospital and bring them with me the following week when we would be there for Shae-Lynne's pre-op. *This was unbelievable.* This meant that I now had to do the two-hour drive the following day to pick up the CT scans at the hospital in Sydney and that basically this had been a wasted trip.

* * *

It was May third. Shae-Lynne would be operated on tomorrow. We had to leave for Halifax this morning to be in time for her pre-op this afternoon. Unfortunately, Michael could not get away from work, so I had to do the four-hour drive alone with Shae-Lynne. Michael would join us Friday evening after work. I was not a big fan of driving long distances. I would usually end up with a migraine and I tend to get sleepy while I drive. I was very nervous about the trip, and perhaps that may have temporarily helped to keep my mind off Shae-Lynne's surgery.

From the beginning of the drive, I had struggled to keep my eyes open. Then about twenty minutes into our drive, I jumped and realized that I had drifted over the yellow line. My eyes had closed. My heart raced and my hands shook. It scared me enough to keep me awake for an hour or so. I felt my eyes getting heavy again and I still had a two-and-a-half-hour drive to reach the hospital. I had to do something. I popped a Bob Seger tape into the cassette deck, turned the sound up and started to sing. I was tapping the wheel and bopping around. I had to stay awake. People passing by must have thought I was a mad woman.

We finally arrived safe and sound at the hospital. My head was beginning to pound, not a good sign. At one point I overheard two nurses talking about Shae-Lynne's upcoming surgery. The nurse looking after us mentioned to the other nurse about Shae-Lynne having a *roux en y* tomorrow. I had to interrupt, "No," I said, "she is having a jejunostomy."

"Oh," the nurse responded, "I thought it was a roux en y."

Now, after all my research and everything I learned, I knew to question her response. When we had originally been discussing the possibility of Shae-Lynne requiring surgery, I had posted a question to the moms on the tube feeding board on-line about jejunostomies and the J-tube in general. I was looking for their experiences and advice. A couple of moms wrote to say that they had no experience with this, but had heard jejunostomies might be dangerous. They knew of a child who had permanent problems because of it. After a few days of reading these posts, another mom e-mailed me privately and told me they were mistaken. It was her son that they were speaking of and he had a roux en y, not a jejunostomy. I was so glad she had contacted me. She went on to explain that the roux en y was cutting the bowel in half and stitching one side to the stomach wall and one to the large intestine. That is what her son had trouble with—not the jejunostomy itself.

At the time I read this I did not pay much attention to it. I assumed her son had other problems that required this surgery and it did not pertain to me. Now our nurse was explaining to the other nurse the roux en y is what they were planning to do to Shae-Lynne. I don't think so. We met with the surgeon to have him clear this up.

"I was under the impression that my daughter was having a jejunostomy performed tomorrow and I heard the nurse say that Shae-Lynne was scheduled for a roux en y. Which are you planning to do?" I asked.

"The surgery we have planned for Shae-Lynne requires cutting the small intestine in half. We will stitch one half to the abdominal wall and a hole will be cut there for the J-tube. The other half, the upper half (duodenum) coming from the stomach will be sutured to the large intestine. This will be permanent and we don't feel it would cause problems down the line." He drew a small diagram for me, to illustrate his point and spoke about it a bit more.

I was angry. This is not what we discussed earlier. I didn't need this long description or diagram. I knew what a roux en y was and I knew what a jejunostomy was. All I wanted to know was which he had planned to do. It was almost as though he was trying to talk over me. Did he think I didn't know the difference and by not using the actual term that I would be okay with it? I felt like he was trying to lead me to believe that this was the only surgery they performed for the J-tube insertion and that what he was describing was a jejunostomy.

With anger and frustration I responded, "Yes, but that is a roux en y. My husband and I agreed to have a jejunostomy, not a roux en y. There is no way I want all that done to my daughter. Go in, make your little hole in her jejunum, put in the tube and get out." Ugh! If I hadn't overheard the nurses' conversation and had not been familiar with the term, I never would have known what they were planning. I could not understand why they would automatically do such a complicated procedure when there was a much simpler alternative.

"We have been shying away from jejunostomies as they have been frequently failing. Too many times a second surgery is needed to perform the roux en y anyway after the jejunostomy fails. We started doing the roux en y in the first place to save the extra surgery. Roux en ys also tend to leak less fluid than the jejunostomy. We feel it is more secure. I would really prefer to do the roux en y, Roni. But, in the end, it is your decision. You and your husband can decide whatever you are more comfortable with."

Now I understood and felt a bit guilty that I had become so angry. However, it did not change the fact that we should have been told this before now. We should have been given the choice to make. I thought this is great; one day before surgery, I am alone, and I have no computer to research this further and I have a huge decision to make. Why didn't they explain this before?

I knew I did not want the roux en y. It would be permanently altering the way Shae-Lynne's body worked and it was much more invasive. It didn't matter that I had heard the horror story about it. But if I did decide to do the jejunostomy, would she require the roux en y eventually? What was I going to do? I asked if I could speak with Michael about it and give our decision tomorrow before surgery. The surgeon said that would be fine.

Now my head was really pounding.

Then off to meet with Dr. Peters, the neurosurgeon again—this time with the CT scans. After looking at the scans, he re-confirmed his previous statement that he was certain the fluid had nothing to do with Shae-Lynne's vomiting. He said that this CT scan looked the same as the original one and although it did show a little extra fluid, it may or may not mean anything. As usual we were left with more questions than answers.

After spending the afternoon in the hospital getting Shae-Lynne ready for the next day's surgery, we were able to go to my friend Cheryl's house and relax. I was really looking forward to seeing her again. Cheryl lived close to the hospital and had welcomed us for the evening. We were in school together since we were six years old and had become very close friends the last couple of years in high school. We had remained close ever since, even though we were now further apart physically.

I needed to relax but most importantly I needed to eat. I hadn't eaten anything all day. I crashed on the couch and Cheryl ordered a pizza. It was a perfect way to end such a stressful day.

Just as we were finishing our pizza, our friend Lisa and my cousin Jennifer came over. Cheryl had planned a small surprise birthday party for Shae-Lynne (who would be turning one on May sixteenth). She pulled a birthday cake out of the fridge that read "Happy Birthday Shae-Lynne." Next out came the ice cream and balloons. I don't think Cheryl knew how much it meant to me. I was so touched that she went to so much trouble on our behalf and even remembered Shae-Lynne's birthday. It was still two weeks away. It was the nicest thing she could've done.

Now it was time to fill Michael in on our day. I called and discussed our options with him. It was difficult to present the facts to him without swaying his opinion. I tried to be as neutral as I could when explaining each procedure. He was adamantly opposed to the roux en y and was furious that they even considered it without telling us. I made sure he understood that the jejunostomy could fail and then Shae-Lynne would need to have the roux en y anyway. It was ultimately decided that we wanted the least invasive thing possible. So we decided on the jejunostomy and we would hope for the best.

* * *

It was nine a.m. as Shae-Lynne and I arrived at the hospital. My stomach was upset. I felt like I was going to throw up and I also felt guilty. Shae-Lynne was happy, playing and smiling. She had no clue about what was about to happen. I felt like a traitor. We made our way to the room that we would be in after the surgery. I plopped our bags down knowing that this would be home for the next week. As I prepared the crib (raising the head and setting up the blankets), the resident surgeon came in with the permission slip for me to sign. She explained the procedure (which I was already familiar with from my research) and the risks involved. She then passed the paper to me. Up until now I was doing okay, a couple stray tears here and there. When she passed me that permission slip, the floodgates opened. I completely fell apart for what would most certainly not be the last time that day. In an attempt to comfort me, she put her arm around me. It did not help. I just needed a minute to compose myself.

I was so angry. If only I were stronger. I felt like such an idiot and maybe a bit guilty. I cried like a baby over what many would consider simple surgery. I knew there were many other kids much sicker than Shae-Lynne. So many other parents making life and death decisions for their children every day. I wondered how they were able to do it. But that was other people and this was *my* baby! How did it come to this? I think if the surgery were being performed to cure Shae-Lynne it would have been easier to accept. However, this day I was giving permission for our daughter to be sliced open, simply to feed her. I did not believe she would be any better after this surgery.

I eventually pulled myself together enough to sign the permission slip and Shae-Lynne and I headed to the operating room waiting area. I sat in the same rocking chair that I had sat in so many months earlier when Michael and I were there for Shae-Lynne's endoscopy. I stared at the same butterfly poster on the wall, wishing that she were simply having another scope test. After what seemed like an eternity, a nurse came to say that they were ready for her. My chest felt as though it were in vice grips, heavy and tight, I could hardly breathe. My knees were weak and wobbling, my stomach hurt and tears began to trickle down my face as I gave Shae-Lynne the biggest hug and kiss I could. I told her I loved her, held her another moment and then reluctantly passed her to the nurse. Immediately she began to scream at the top of her lungs and desperately tried to wiggle her way back to me with her arms reaching for me, as she did whenever anyone else held her. My heart was breaking. All I wanted to do was knock out the nurse, grab Shae-Lynne and run away as fast as I could. This was agonizing. Shae-Lynne screamed all the way down the hall and I sat in *my* chair and cried. I pictured her being taken to this roomful of strangers, kicking, screaming and terrified, while they held her down to get an IV in her tiny arm. Then I was picturing her sedated little body lying lifeless on the operating table bed while they sliced her stomach.

I can't do this. I have to stop thinking about it. Quickly I decided I did not want to sit here for the next two hours in hysterics while others walked by and watched. I needed to get away and do something constructive. I headed up to Shae-Lynne's room in an attempt to keep busy. I called to have the phone hooked up, called to get a parking pass, called my mom, unpacked all of Shae-Lynne's toys and books and carefully arranged them around her crib. I had to try to keep my mind off what was happening to her.

With all that done I took out the copy of Bernie Siegel, MD's book *Peace, Love & Healing* that Mom bought for me. This was the first time I had any time to myself so I looked forward to reading it. I was so glad I brought it. I love reading his work. It was so refreshing to find a doctor who became so involved in his patients and cared so much for people. Some of the people he wrote about are truly inspiring. It was a perfect way to keep occupied, although as I read, my mind would wander back to Shae-Lynne's surgery.

At last they called from surgery that Shae-Lynne was waking and I could go down to the recovery area to see her. I walked in, washed my hands, and scanned the room as I had done so many months earlier. A nurse was wheeling a bed toward me. There was Shae-Lynne, so tiny, so still. Her sweet face wasn't as swollen as it was when she had her scope done. She looked a little better to me this time, although there were more tubes attached to her. There was an IV in her hand, which would be her nutrition for the next few days. An extra IV was placed in one foot with nothing attached to it, just in case the one in her hand came out. Shae-Lynne also had a catheter to collect urine. They had placed a bandage type thing on her toe for the oxygen monitor.

The NG tube was still in Shae-Lynne's nose. I was so disappointed to see it there as I thought it would be gone by now. Her nurse explained that they would use it to drain Shae-Lynne's stomach juices and acids for the next few days until she healed. They didn't want anything going into her bowel just yet. I gritted my teeth and agreed that it made sense. It sickened me to see Shae-Lynne like this. No wonder she was so terrified of people.

Shae-Lynne started to open her eyes slightly, and they caught mine. She cried and cried until I made the nurse let me hold her. Initially, when the nurse moved her, she cried harder. I felt badly for having her moved and possibly causing discomfort. However, as soon as I put her in my arms and snuggled my head next to hers, she calmed down and began to fall back to sleep. I was extremely uncomfortable and began to get a headache. I didn't care, Shae-Lynne was in my arms and she was content. That was all that mattered. After a few minutes of peaceful sleep, she jerked and cried out as if she had gotten a sharp jolt of pain. This continued every couple minutes and I repeatedly insisted that the nurse do something to help her. Since Shae-Lynne's heart rate was extremely high, the nurse eventually agreed to increase her intake of morphine. This seemed to settle Shae-Lynne.

After two hours in the recovery room we were allowed to go back up to our room. My head was pounding more by the minute. It was getting difficult to move and close to migraine status. I was determined to ignore the pain. Shae-Lynne needed me and was surely feeling worse than I. I would just sit, relax, and rock us both to sleep. I hoped that would make me feel better. After an hour had passed, Shae-Lynne seemed comfortable and I dozed off for a short time. Unfortunately, I was feeling worse. A nurse came in and I asked for a cot and help to get Shae-Lynne into her crib. I set the cot up beside the crib and lay down. By now Shae-Lynne was awake and not at all pleased with her situation. I turned cartoons on to distract her so I could lie quietly. The more I moved the worse I felt. I was so furious with myself. I was a miserable excuse for a mother. I wasn't about to ask the nurse for anything to relieve the pain because then she would know what a crummy mother I was. If only Michael would get here so I could sleep for an hour.

By the time Michael arrived I was throwing up. The migraine was beyond the point of sleeping it off. Shortly after Michael arrived, Cheryl came to visit. I sent her out to the drug store for me. Gravol, Tylenol, Aspirin and Advil—that was her mission. I took one of each and went to sleep for an hour. Thankfully, when I woke up my pain had eased enough so that I wasn't throwing up anymore.

I awoke to find Shae-Lynne crying a lot and visibly uncomfortable. Michael was unable to comfort her so I got up and lay my head down beside hers in the crib. It relaxed Shae-Lynne somewhat, but I could tell she was still miserable. All of a sudden she gagged and her lips were doing her patented pre-puke wiggling. I didn't even reach for a towel. Not only was there no food in her stomach, it's being pumped of all its gastric juices. No way, she's not going to puke. Actually, I wondered why she was even gagging. A second later I wished I had instinctively grabbed a towel, as Shae-Lynne threw up all over herself. *How can that be?* "Damn it, what do we have to do to make this kid quit puking?"

The next day the nurse came in to change Shae-Lynne's dressing. She told me that I should watch her so that on the following day I could do it by myself. Huh, I don't think so. I wasn't prepared to look at the surgery site yet. I was definitely not going to watch her change the dressing, nor would I be ready to do it myself the next day. I had to work my way into it slowly. When I was ready. After all, what was the rush, we would be there for the next few days so I had time.

It was so nice having Michael with me now. Over the next two days I tried to get out as much as I could because I knew that once he went home on Sunday, I wouldn't be able to leave Shae-Lynne's room until her suction tube was removed (it was attached to the wall beside the crib). Once that was out I could at least put her in the stroller and wheel the IV stand along with us. I wouldn't be leaving the hospital again though until Shae-Lynne was discharged. I went for a walk and took a drive to the mall on Saturday afternoon for two hours. That was my break and it would have to last me all week.

The next day when the nurse came in to change the dressing, I stood by the crib and took a couple of peaks at it. The first time I looked at it I got weak and had to sit down. I couldn't look at it for long but I was just pleased that I could bring myself to even get near it. I hated it. My perfect little angel had a big rubber hose sticking out of the side of her belly. It looked like something you'd see in a science-fiction movie. It wasn't really gross at all. In fact, the site was very clean and neat with perfect pink skin next to the catheter (that is the technical term, not hose). It was just so foreign.

Michael headed for home later Sunday afternoon. I hated to see him go and I could tell he did not want to leave us. I would have been lonely and bored if not for the great couple who shared our room. Their eight-year-old daughter had come in sometime Friday evening and had her appendix out that same night. They were very friendly. All the times Shae-Lynne had been in a hospital the past year this was the first time she had to share a room. I really got lucky, and was actually glad for their company.

Shae-Lynne continued to throw up. Although I asked repeatedly how that could be possible when her stomach was being suctioned. I was dismissed, ignored and never got an answer. One afternoon during mid-week, Shae-Lynne had another very bad throw-up episode and stopped breathing again.

Stephen (the little girl's dad) went charging out of the room to find a nurse. Thankfully, just as they were coming back into the room, Shae-Lynne started to breathe.

The week went by quickly. Each day I was able to look at Shae-Lynne's site a bit more and got closer to it than the day before. Just a few days before Shae-Lynne was to be released, the surgeon, while doing his rounds, gave the okay to take out the NG tube. The minute he left the room, I loosened the tape on her face and pulled out her nasal tube for the last time. I wasn't about to wait all day for the nurse to come in and do it. As I removed the tube I was left with an almost bittersweet feeling. I was so glad to see Shae-Lynne's beautiful face. However, the tube had been such a big part of who she was for the majority of her short life—it was odd but in some bizarre way I thought I might miss it. Now that her NG tube was out she was no longer hooked to the suction on the wall. I was able to take her away from our room for walks in the stroller. She was getting so very restless stuck in the crib every day. She was desperately trying to get up and walk all the time. It was a constant struggle every day to keep her off her feet—as the spare IV was still in her foot.

One evening a volunteer came into our room and told us about the playroom at the end of the hall. I took Shae-Lynne down to play for a while. As I watched the volunteers, I couldn't help but think what great people they were for taking time out of their day to spend with these kids. Most people never give sick kids a second thought. I know I didn't until I had one. I wondered if these volunteers realized what a difference they were making and the joy they brought to these little patients, as well as their parents.

* * *

We were able to leave the hospital on Friday. It was exactly one week after Shae-Lynne's surgery and again I had to drive the four hours home alone. We made it safe and sound. Shae-Lynne was so glad to see Daddy, as was I.

The pressure was on us for the first couple of weeks. We were told that if the tube accidentally pulled out in the first six weeks, it would have to be surgically re-inserted.

It was now June. Shae-Lynne was thirteen months old, weighed sixteen and a half pounds (the size of an average six-month-old). Her vomiting had lessened considerably after the surgery, and was now down to two or three a day. We thought this was wonderful.

Our biggest problem now was her fear. Shae-Lynne feared everything and everyone. She appeared traumatized by both the surgery and hospital stay. She was welded to me more than usual and would not even let me leave the room or leave her sight for one second. If it appeared that I was getting up to leave the room, she screamed. It didn't even matter if Daddy was still with her. Most days she only wanted to sit in my lap for long periods of time and be cuddled. By now Shae-Lynne had stopped sleeping in her crib. She would wake screaming, as if having a nightmare, and wouldn't go back to sleep unless she was in our bed, beside me or in my lap. This happened at naptime as well as through the night. She had always been excessively attached to me; however, this was ridiculous. I never really had a life prior to the surgery but now I couldn't even walk freely through the house. I was tired, frustrated, and in desperate need of alone time.

* * *

Everything about Shae-Lynne had to be handled differently than with a normal baby. Screaming and getting upset made Shae-Lynne throw up. With the amount of throwing up she had done the past year we walked on eggshells. We had to keep her from screaming to prevent as many throw ups as possible. If the only thing that was going to help her deal with the pain and puking was Mommy cuddling her, then that was what she was going to get.

Sometimes I felt as though I coddled her a little too much, and so did many other people. But this beautiful little girl has felt pain that I cannot imagine every single day of her short life. The only thing I can do is make sure Mommy is always there when she is needed. Maybe I do coddle her too much. Maybe I don't. All I know is that I am doing the best that I can for her under very difficult circumstances.

In August, Mom came for another visit. Shae-Lynne was ever so slowly beginning to adjust to people. She was very good with my mom. Shae-Lynne let Mom hold her a few times and they held hands and walked along the boardwalk looking at the boats. I was thrilled that they had bonded as before. A couple of days before Mom was to leave for home Shae-Lynne started to throw up more frequently. Overall she just seemed miserable most of the day and night. I didn't think too much of it and chalked it up to the heat. I assumed things would improve. They didn't. By the time my mom left Shae-Lynne was getting worse every day.

Shae-Lynne was up all night, every night, crying and throwing up. Her days were a nightmare. It started when she woke; puke after puke after puke, most not even an hour apart. When she wasn't throwing up, all she did was lie in my lap and whimper.

* * *

8:30 a.m. and Shae Lynne is starting to stir. I awaken, as usual. I'm so tired I can barely open my eyes and yet somehow I do. I roll over to look at her face, and wonder if she is about to throw up again. For sure, her mouth is wiggling and she's beginning to whine and cry. *Here we go again*, I think to myself with a sigh of irritation. This is how our day had started every single morning for the past two weeks or more. I reach for a towel and as we have done so many times, Shae-Lynne begins to vomit and I attempt to comfort her and clean her up.

It's 9:15 a.m. before Shae-Lynne finishes vomiting and settles down enough so that we can get up and dress. I carry her downstairs and lay her on her changing pad propped up on the pillows we have always kept underneath it.

As I start to change her diaper she begins to gag. Ugh, I am so sick of this I just want to scream! *Not again, not again, please not again*, I pray to myself. She proceeds with her throwing up. Ten minutes later she settles down again. I get her dressed for the day. She appears to be feeling okay so I put her on the floor to play.

Since Shae-Lynne loves to stand and is able to walk some on her own, we bought her a play table with activities on the top. She seemed to be having a wonderful time, cruising around the table and entertaining herself with noises and such. Within five to ten minutes, for no apparent reason she begins to scream, a loud, high-pitched scream of pain. She grabs at her belly and chest, definitely in discomfort of some sort. I pick her up and we sit in the recliner. The cuddling seems to make her feel a little better. We sit together for an hour or more as she whines and cries on and off and throws up a couple of more times. Every so often I try to put her down to play; however, she screams. She leaves her legs limp so as not to be able to stand.

Something is most definitely bothering her. We sit until she is ready to play again. I've become very good at being able to tell the difference between her looking for attention and when she is truly feeling horrible. When she is feeling this badly, everything else gets put on hold for as long as she needs me.

Eventually she gets wiggly and wants down so I put her on the floor to play again. Ten minutes or more pass, Shae-Lynne stops what she is doing and emits more high-pitched screams. Once more I pick her up and we sit together in the chair as I try to settle her and keep her from throwing up. Again we sit for over an hour with the intermittent cries. She is so exhausted from all the throwing up that she has no energy left to get up and be active. When she decides to play again, she lets me know by trying to wiggle to the floor. Over and over, all day this is repeated. She plays for about ten minutes and then sits and cries, throws up and whimpers for an hour or more.

I try my best to get through every day by keeping her as comfortable as possible. By now I know that she has good spells and bad spells. The reflux moms I know refer to this as the so-called "reflux roller coaster." Surely she will come around soon and improve. I hold onto this hope every morning as the day begins. I would convince myself that today would be a better day and if it wasn't I would look forward to tomorrow.

This was to be our new routine for over two weeks before I couldn't take it anymore and called Dr. Andrews. Perhaps he could increase her Losec now that she's a little older. Yes, he said to double it. I couldn't believe it, double it just like that? Of course I was willing to try anything at that point. So, I increased her daily dose from ten mgs to twenty mgs. Now at fifteen months and still the same sixteen and a half pounds as a few months ago, Shae-Lynne was on an adult dose of this medication. Unfortunately, it did not help.

My next thought was to switch her formula. I had been doing that frequently before her surgery and it seemed to help. Since her surgery I hadn't switched it at all because until now she had been doing well. First I tried Compleat Pediatric, as she had done well on that before. I was a little nervous to put Shae-Lynne on it now though because of its intact proteins. The Neocate (which she was currently taking) was completely broken down so that her body didn't have to do much to absorb it. I had gotten her rate (amount of formula she was able to ingest) per hour up pretty high. I feared that if I introduced a complete protein at such a high rate she would not be able to tolerate it, as it would take too long to digest.

I don't know if I was right or not but Shae-Lynne certainly didn't tolerate the Compleat this time around. Within twenty minutes of starting her on the Compleat she began to vomit up much more frequently. I didn't think it was possible but about every half hour or so for almost four hours she threw up. It was insufferable. After about four hours I couldn't watch her like that anymore and stopped the Compleat. She always seemed to feel much better on water and Pedialyte so for a few hours I gave her that just to give her a break. I guess it was back to the Neocate.

The next day I called the nutritionist at Children's Hospital. She had previously suggested I try Vivonex Pediatric (an amino acid based formula similar to Neocate). Up until now I had been a bit skeptical because Shae-Lynne had begun to react so poorly to the regular Vivonex last spring. I was desperate though. This time the nutritionist felt there wasn't much point in trying the Vivonex Pediatric, as it was so similar to the Neocate. I insisted (we had to try something) and since she had no better ideas she sent me some to try.

It came within two days and with my fingers crossed I mixed it and put it into Shae-Lynne's bag. Again, within twenty minutes she was throwing up more than ever. This time she threw up almost non-stop for about four hours, until I shut it off. I stopped the formula and again gave her water and Pedialyte.

By now I'm at my wit's end. I can't watch her like this anymore. Every time I think she can't possibly get any worse—she does. Shae-Lynne had never been this bad. Feeding her was torture. I knew by feeding her that I was the one making her so incredibly sick. I also knew that she needed the calories and nutrition to live. But what kind of quality of life is this for her? Every few days I diluted her formula somewhat with water or Pedialyte for a few hours just to help her feel a little better. It always made a big difference. Then I'd feel guilty all day knowing I was not providing Shae-Lynne with the proper nutrition. I had given up on her gaining any weight at this point. I just needed to find a delicate balance between keeping her nourished and not crying and throwing up twenty times a day.

It was over three weeks, probably more like four, that Shae-Lynne had been like this, and it was taking its toll on her. Not to mention me. I broke down and called to make an appointment with Dr. Andrews. His secretary squeezed us in the next day.

We walked into Dr. Andrews' office and sat on the big couch against the back wall as we had so many other times. Shae-Lynne sat on my lap snuggled into my arms, listless, whimpering and miserable. She had thrown up on her blouse on the way to the appointment and I was just noticing some I missed when cleaning her. She proceeded to throw up two more times in the short time we were in his office, while I continued to explain this is the way it had been going the past few weeks. I really didn't have to say much though, Dr. Andrews could now see for himself.

"The poor little thing. She can't go on like this," he said with sadness in his eyes, "and neither can you," he continued as he glanced at me. My fatigue was apparent.

When Shae-Lynne was initially diagnosed with reflux, I insisted the doctors had to have missed something. I did not believe that something so common and harmless could be the cause of all the pain and suffering Shae-Lynne had endured since birth. When I began my research and found there were so many other kids going through hell because of reflux, I started to understand. Reflux could very well be the cause.

Dr. Andrews was now a little skeptical himself as he sat and watched. He just sat for a few moments watching Shae-Lynne, her file on his lap. The tip of a pen in his mouth, he looked a bit perplexed and deep in thought. We sat in silence for what seemed like an eternity before he finally spoke. "I just can't help but think there's something else going on here that we've missed." Great, I thought, just when I finally accept this reflux theory.

"I think we should have another CT scan done and in the meantime, I'm going to see if I can get the radiologist in Halifax to look at her previous CT scans again. Just give me a minute here." He slid his chair over to his desk and picked up the phone.

After he hung up, I tried to make him understand it was the food that made Shae-Lynne sick. Maybe a little for my own benefit, if it was food making her sick then it wasn't something neurological. But the fact was, the less food Shae-Lynne got the better she was.

"Why don't we keep her again for the weekend and try a central line for a couple days. That will give her digestive system a break and hopefully help her feel a little better for a while. I also think it will give us some insight as to whether it's neurological or gastrointestinal. I mean if she still vomits then we can be pretty certain it's neurological; however, if the TPN stops the vomiting, it is likely to be gastrointestinal, right?" He waited for my response.

I sat in silence. On the drive to our appointment I was fearful Dr. Andrews might suggest TPN. I had read online of a few women whose children were sent home totally TPN fed and I was really afraid it might be coming to that with Shae-Lynne. It's not as if we had any formula options left and it didn't matter anyway, she clearly wasn't tolerating any kind of feeding. But I kept coming back to the fact she does do well for awhile.

I sighed. "Oh, I don't know if I can put Shae-Lynne through another hospital stay. She is so terrified of people as it is." I told him a little about her anxiety around other people and how it always got worse after hospitalization.

"I understand your fears. It's up to you." He is such a nice man and I knew he wanted to help as much as I wanted him to.

I thought back to the first time that he mentioned the possibility of tube feeding "for the weekend" and look where we are now. I pictured the central line going in for the TPN and us going home indefinitely on TPN, I couldn't handle that. Of course, I didn't think I could handle tube feeding and yet somehow I was.

It was very difficult for me to know what to do. I wanted to do what was best for Shae-Lynne. Unfortunately, I didn't know what that was. Every other time Dr. Andrews wanted to admit her I went along with it and let him do what he thought was best. Every hospital stay thus far had left Shae-Lynne more frightened than the last. She had gotten to the point that she cried if someone looked at her. Her fear is almost as heartbreaking to me as the condition of her health. The other thing that went through my mind was that following her previous surgery she had TPN for a few days while she healed. However, she still continued to vomit, albeit not nearly as much as before.

After thinking of the pros and cons I gave Dr. Andrews my opinion. "I am not convinced that anything would be accomplished by Shae-Lynne being admitted." I was also thinking, could we survive any longer with how sick Shae-Lynne was? I brought up these points to Dr. Andrews and since he was still waiting to hear from the neurology department at Children's Hospital, together we decided to wait.

On the hour drive home Shae-Lynne threw up three times and cried most of the way. I had to stop several times to calm her. I felt sick inside as I was beginning to think I had made the wrong choice. Perhaps I should have agreed to the TPN. When I arrived home I called Dr. Andrews back to get the okay to dilute the formula to half strength for the weekend. He said that would be fine and he would call back the first of the week.

Almost immediately after diluting the formula Shae-Lynne improved and the vomiting decreased. By the beginning of the week she was only throwing up about a half dozen times a day. She also spent more time playing. I started very slowly increasing the strength of her formula again, until she was up to twenty-two calories per ounce. This still was not full strength; however, when I went higher the vomiting resumed. We settled for that and left her feed running for a couple of extra hours to make up the difference.

Now that Shae-Lynne had magically improved on her own, I was so grateful that I decided against admitting her for the weekend to try the TPN as Dr. Andrews had suggested. I followed my gut feeling and finally made a good decision. I had pictured them holding Shae-Lynne down to get the IV in place and it felt so good to know that I didn't put her through that needlessly.

By this time the surgical site had healed enough so that Shae-Lynne could have a button inserted and the catheter removed. A button would make her site much easier to manage and more comfortable. The appointment was scheduled for a Friday and Michael took the day off work to come with us on the four-hour drive to Children's Hospital. After the long drive by myself for her surgery I swore I wasn't doing that again. This would be a day surgery procedure. After they had finished and Shae-Lynne woke enough, I was given a quick lesson on how to use the button and off we went for home.

The button is a little plastic device that sits relatively flat against the surface of the stomach. It has a small hole with a one-way valve that goes into the stomach (or in Shae-Lynne's case her jejunum). There is an extension connecting tube that you insert into the button and the feeding bag plugs into the extension tubing. When Shae-Lynne is not being fed the extension tube can be removed leaving only the small plastic button.

As soon as we arrived home the dressing had to be changed. Shae-Lynne's site had leaked through the gauze the nurses had applied. Her belly looked a little red and irritated so I changed the gauze and rubbed a little petroleum jelly around the site to protect it against the acid that was leaking out. From what I understand, some sites leak a little, some leak a lot and some don't leak at all. The luck of the draw I guess. Since it is acid that leaks out, it can irritate and burn the skin with which it comes in contact. Shae-Lynne's site had always leaked some. Not a lot but enough that I always kept gauze on it. Before the button we did not have a problem with her getting burned because of the device that we used to keep the foley catheter in place. It had a round, rather large base that stuck to her stomach, protecting it against leakage. Now that it was gone her belly looked a little red.

Within a few hours I had to change the dressing again. Poor Shae-Lynne, her stomach was still red so I sloughed on more petroleum jelly and hoped for the best. This continued through the next day and night. I knew when it was time to change the gauze, as Shae-Lynne would begin to cry and rub her belly. By the time evening came I knew I would need to get something stronger than Vaseline. Unfortunately, the drug store didn't open until 2:00 p.m. the next day.

Shae-Lynne was up throughout the night. She cried and rubbed her belly in spite of how often I changed her dressing. By morning the gauze was soaked and her belly was red. She had quite a severe looking rash. As we waited for the drug store to open, I continued to change her dressing and put as much Vaseline on the site as possible. It was useless though, as acid was literally pouring out of her site. It ate right through the Vaseline and was getting worse. The acid leaking out onto Shae-Lynne's skin that was already irritated from acid was now blistering her sensitive skin. She was miserable. She cried and rubbed her stomach so hard I thought for sure she was going to pop the button. Two o'clock could not come fast enough. I picked up some zinc cream and some duoderm (a thin protective tape that has a healing agent). The duoderm made a big difference. She finally got some relief, but it was very difficult to remove. After a couple of days, the acid would eat away at the duoderm and if it wasn't changed Shae-Lynne was back to getting burned again. I spoke with one of the nurses at Children's Hospital and she suggested a cream called Proshield that is made for G- and J-tube sites that leak. She also suggested sprinkling a powder called Stomadhesive onto the site before applying the duoderm; she thought that would make it easier to get off.

Eventually we received a call to have Shae-Lynne's CT scan repeated as Dr. Andrews had requested in August. We took it to Dr. Peters, Shae-Lynne's neurologist at Children's Hospital, on the same day she had her GI check up. Dr. Clements, the GI, said the usual—nothing. He weighed her and measured her. That was about it. I brought him up-to-date: Shae-Lynne was doing better now but that August had been hell. He had no explanation. He passed the buck and said perhaps Dr. Peters could shed some light on things when we saw him in a few minutes. He could do nothing more, perhaps her problem was neurological.

We headed up to neurology where again, there were no answers. Dr. Peters reaffirmed his previous diagnosis. He was convinced that Shae-Lynne's vomiting was not related to anything neurological. Although the CT scans were slightly abnormal it may not mean anything. Only time would tell.

"What are we supposed to do now? Do we just continue like this and let Shae-Lynne live her life throwing up a few times a day and accept that? She may be doing better now only as compared to before. Would you want to throw up a few times a day every day? Someone has to be able to do something." I was exasperated. "GI says they can't do anything else, maybe you can offer some answers. You say you can't do anything, just wait it out."

I described how Shae-Lynne throws up, hoping he would understand. It is definitely different, not spit up like most people assume. Determined for an answer, I was not backing down. "She throws her guts up as though she has food poisoning or the stomach flu. It's so hard on her," I told him.

His only suggestion was to tape it and send a copy to him. Perhaps if he saw her in action it may help. So we left his office and headed for home again, very disappointed.

CHAPTER EIGHT

IN CLOSING

This is where we stand now. I have since sent the tape of Shae-Lynne vomiting to Dr. Peters. He watched it with Dr. Clements and the entire pediatric department. They ordered a few tests, all of which came back normal and now they have nothing left to say. So, we plug along with the tube feeds and vomiting. That's reflux life!

Shae-Lynne at eighteen months and just over seventeen pounds has no interest in eating at all. She doesn't know how and doesn't know why she should eat. It is completely foreign to her. She is on twenty-hour-a-day continuous feeds so there is no hope of her learning what an appetite is any time soon. If she ever gains enough weight to be able to spare a few pounds we will attempt cutting back her tube feeds enough to give her an appetite so she will learn why she has to eat.

After eighteen months of watching Shae-Lynne suffer, I must admit that getting her to eat is not my top priority. So many times in the days and weeks following Shae-Lynne's birth, our lives revolved around her eating. I can't even count the number of times I begged her, "Please, please, please eat!" Now all I care about is that she is happy and feeling good. The eating will come, someday, when she is ready.

Shae-Lynne's site continues to leak a lot more than I would like, but as with everything else I have learned to adapt. My goal is to prevent burns and to keep the redness and pain to a minimum. I have accepted the fact that her site is probably always going to be a little red and irritated with the amount that Shae-Lynne leaks.

I'm sure we will be dealing with some degree of health, feeding and speech issues for years to come. Right now the surgeon confirms Shae-Lynne is not a good candidate for the fundoplication and that's fine by me. Michael and I are not willing to take a chance on it anyway. Perhaps that will change once Shae-Lynne is old enough to tell us how much she hurts, but hopefully by then she won't hurt so much.

It is because of Shae-Lynne's good spells—like she is having now—that we are able to survive her not-so-good spells. I know that at any time she could start with a bad streak again but I also know that it won't last forever. I have succumbed to the fact that I will probably never know why she has good spells and bad spells. Frankly, I'm far too weary to keep trying to figure it out.

Writing Shae-Lynne's story has been exceptionally difficult for me. It would not have been completed if not for my mother. Only through her determination and persistence (that's a nice way to say nagging) did I get this finished. I have been very torn in writing this, perhaps that is part of why it was so difficult.

There is a huge part of me that does not want our lives made so public. I also realize that there are so many children much sicker than Shae-Lynne with terminal diseases, debilitating disorders and severe mental and physical impairments. There are even kids with reflux who are sicker than Shae-Lynne. I don't want to minimize their suffering. Also bothering me is that I am not a writer and was therefore fearful that I would not be able to do justice to this disease. I was concerned that I would not do a good job getting across how serious infant GERD is.

But an even bigger part of me knows that this needs to be done. I can't even begin to count the number of moms that have e-mailed me after finding Shae-Lynne's website. Their gratitude for finding such a site and for the information provided is overwhelming. They are so grateful to find someone who understands, and they are all so desperate to help their kids. Here are just a few of the hundreds of e-mails I have received.

* * *

My son is eight and has a long painful history with reflux. We have been through tons of doctors and have also tried alternative practitioners all with only partial relief. As a baby he was diagnosed as having reflux 75% of the time and it still plagues him. He is eight, but appears more like a five-year-old. Recently he has stopped eating dinner, being only too aware of the painful consequences. I am scared and feel there is so little hope!

He obviously has a severe case. I hope your little one does better than that. I'm not even sure why I am writing, just that I feel so alone with this and frustrated. His pediatrician says, "That is Jimmy" and "Give him Maalox or Mylanta before a meal."

My husband and I are small. I hate the possibility of him being even smaller because he doesn't get the nutrition he needs. Jimmy has learning disabilities as well and I can't help but wonder if these come from lack of adequate nutrition.

As you said, medical science has so few answers and doesn't even seem to want to ask the questions.

Please let me know if you hear of anything that seems to improve the condition.

* * *

I read the heartbreaking story of your daughter and it particularly touched me since my daughter was just diagnosed with GERD. She is ten weeks old, but she was born five weeks early. From the beginning she had problems eating and had to stay one week in the hospital. Thankfully she has been gaining weight, but she is now on medications (Prevacid and Reglan). The problem seems to be getting worse instead of better and it is very discouraging. I have spent hours crying while trying to feed her. It takes her an hour to get about three ounces down. Then she usually throws it all back up.

This week we see the doctor and I am going to ask for a referral to a pediatric GI specialist to see if they can be of help. The scariest part to me is the risk of aspiration, because I have caught her gagging and choking several times. I am so scared that something is going to happen to her as a result of this reflux. I feel like I cannot enjoy our time together, because I spend so much of it worrying about her. Right now I am planning to make major lifestyle changes in order to care for her. My husband and I are considering moving in with my parents just so she can have 24-hour care. I do hope that doctors will one day find a cure for this and give parents a viable solution. I too have been told that I have to just left her outgrow it, while in the meanwhile she could suffer from SIDS or any other number of life-threatening complications. The "just wait it out" routine does not satisfy me. Good luck to you and if you can offer any sources that might be a support for my daughter and I please forward them.

* * *

Wow! I cannot believe there are other parents that have gone through the same thing we are going through. I just visited Shae's website. It was almost like reading my own thoughts on the screen.

One of my twins, Trent, has had severe eating problems since birth. His growth curve is almost identical to Shae's. He is now 14 months old and weighs 14 pounds. His twin brother weighs 26 pounds.

No one I talk to understands the frustration and helplessness I go through on a daily basis with Trent. I know he is uncomfortable, hungry and confused and I can't do anything about it.

All the doctors I talk to act as though it is something I am doing wrong. I try every suggestion they have and everyone I can think of or find elsewhere, but none work. Trent has not been on a NG tube since he was 10 weeks old (that's when he was released from the hospital). I have often wished the doctors would allow us to have one so we could get some nutrition in him.

Trent also has developmental delays, speech difficulties, oral sensitivities, and delayed gastric emptying time.

* * *

I want to thank you. I have a two-year-old little girl. She has had severe GERD since birth and has been in circles and circles and circles with the doctors and specialists. However, my daughter is special because she has no pain, no discomfort or anything but VOMITING, VOMITING and more VOMITING. That's why she has had so much trouble being diagnosed. I have searched and searched for answers. My daughter has just gone through her second surgery to dilate her esophagus with no luck. The acid refluxing has caused a stricture (which is closure of her esophagus), which allows her to only take in liquids, if we are lucky. It is a very long story and I would love to tell you all about it.

The reason why I am writing today is to say thank you! The doctors make you feel stupid for being frustrated and confused. I am worn out with doctor visits, hospital stays and surgeries. It is refreshing to know I am not alone. I am the only person I know that is going through this. I have checked with the hospital for support groups with no luck.

* * *

I found your site to be such a blessing. 80% of what I learned, my doctor hadn't told me. My nine-month-old is on Zantac, and doing much better. He still gets up one to four times a night though seeming uncomfortable. I usually nurse him, and he goes back to sleep. Keeping him upright after a meal isn't possible at night. We both need to be sleeping all night. Do children with this disorder generally have trouble sleeping? He falls asleep easily for naps, and when we put him down for the night, but will wake up a few hours later. Frequent ear infections are also a problem. The head of his bed is raised a couple inches, but if I go higher, he ends up rolling sideways, or some other direction. Do you have any good advice? Thanks.

* * *

Thank you for your work on your website. I am browsing the Internet trying to find some possible answers for my own little baby who is four and a half months old. She's had acid reflux since birth, and she is in pain a lot. She has many of the symptoms that you listed, and I am afraid for her, she is getting worse, not better. The one thing that makes her look like everything's okay is that she has gained weight well until now. She had the Upper GI done to determine, that yes, she has reflux. Now she chokes and sputters a lot, but doesn't throw up as much. She isn't eating much anymore and when she does, she pops off (I am still nursing her), and she screams and arches her back. Food is hurting her, or the feeding process or something. She just screams a lot now. She is also very "mucousy" since birth, always snotty and goopy and choking and retching. We don't get much sleep at night anymore.

It feels so good to just write what's going on and get the thoughts out in print, so I can see that they do add up to something. I hope that consistency with her medications (Zantac and Reglan) will help improve her tummy and her digestion. Hopefully something good happens before I dry up and have to quit nursing. My situation is so small compared to yours. I am sorry for what you have had to go through.

* * *

Still don't believe how serious this disease is? Don't take our word for it, read a few of the excerpts quoted from *Reflux Digest*, Vol 7, No 2, June 2003. Beth Anderson, Executive Director and founder of Pediatric/Adolescent Gastroesophageal Reflux Association and Jan Burns, M.Ed., Associate Director recently testified before the U.S. House of Representatives, Appropriations Committee.

Jan states: "I have two children with reflux, Jenna and Rebecca. Rebecca has severe asthma and lung damage from her reflux." She then holds up Rebecca's overnight bag full of medication and feeding pump. "She has had numerous surgeries and as many as fifty clinic visits and seventy-five prescription refills in a year. She is cared for by a team of ten medical specialists. Rebecca has a Section 504 plan and nursing plan at school and she often receives home tutoring from the public school because she misses 20-30 days of school in a calendar year. On the days when she can attend school she has to take a snack and a lunch of special foods that she's allowed to eat during the class if she needs to.

"Before Rebecca was born, I had successfully raised two other children and had a Master's degree in early intervention with thirteen years of experience. But, even a medical degree couldn't have prepared me for the sleep deprivation and the 24/7 intensive care parenting required to care for such a critically ill child."

Beth begins her speech with, "Acid reflux in kids is both more painful and more dangerous than it is for adults. The acid can melt tooth enamel, put holes in the esophageal lining, cause asthma, sinus infections, ear infections, pneumonia and it can even lead to Sudden Infant Death. One of our babies choked and died in his mother's arms—looking into her eyes for help.

"The stress on our family was pretty typical. When my daughter Katie was a baby, her care left me dangerously exhausted. We sent her poor three-year-old brother to daycare because I wasn't even capable of carrying on a conversation with him. My breaking point came one day when Katie screamed all the way to the pharmacy, she screamed all the way home and then she spilled her medicine as I was opening it. I lost it. I walked out of the house, down the street and I gave my baby away to the first person I saw. I didn't know the women's name and it didn't matter. At that point anybody was a better mother than me. I came back an hour later and that wonderful woman became my best friend."

The written testimony clearly illustrates the message we are trying to get across. "GERD in adults can be a mild annoyance but it can also lead to adenocarcinoma, which is increasing in frequency. This type of esophageal cancer has a very low survival rate. Many adults who end up in the emergency room for investigation of a possible heart attack are actually suffering from their first attack of GERD. When new drugs are developed for GERD, they automatically become 'blockbusters' (annual sales over a billion dollars) because sufferers are always seeking a better level of relief. The most popular drug for GERD is the top-selling medication of all time with sales of $2.3 billion in 1999.

"GERD in adults can be a very expensive disease leading to many doctors visits, many lost workdays and the use of very expensive medications. The burden of the disease for adults in the US is estimated at $9.3 billion in direct costs alone, double that of colon cancer.

"Ten years ago, GERD in children was considered very rare. However, recent small studies show that 5 to 8 percent of otherwise healthy children have significant symptoms of GERD, but only a small fraction are receiving any treatment at all. These statistics may be low as parents are unfamiliar with pediatric GERD and may not report the symptoms to the doctor. One pediatric gastroenterologist predicted ten years ago that forming PAGER was pointless and we would never find ten other families in the DC area. Not only is pediatric GERD now considered one of the most common childhood ailments, in the Washington DC area it has become a household word. PAGER has thousands of members worldwide, and our web site, www.reflux.org, receives 50,000 hits per month.

"The rate at which pediatric GERD is being diagnosed has increased dramatically, yet pediatric gastroenterologists still suspect that a larger proportion of children suffering from GERD are not properly diagnosed. They are still seeing far too many children who have extremely serious health problems due to GERD that was not recognized by pediatricians. Better awareness and earlier diagnosis should be reducing the number of hospitalizations, yet one recent study demonstrated a twenty-fold increase in pediatric GERD hospitalization between 1971 and 1995. Surgery to correct pediatric GERD is not always effective and is reserved for severe cases, yet it is the third most common surgery in children. There has also been a 600 percent increase in GI medications given to children in recent years. In addition, the incidence of asthma and allergies in children both appear to be on the rise. These diseases are very closely related to GERD with many unfortunate patients suffering from all three conditions. We do know that the actual incidence of GERD in adults has been rising dramatically in the past few decades.

"PAGER refers to caring for a child with GERD as '24-hour intensive care parenting,' with parents often stressed to the breaking point. Many of our members have been diagnosed with clinical depression, and some have even been diagnosed with sleep deprivation psychosis. Most of our members say that caring for a child with GERD is the most difficult thing they have ever dealt with, and many decide not to have additional children for fear of having another child GERD.

"Babies and toddlers with GERD require an extraordinary level of care and with few exceptions their mothers are forced to quit work. Our teens have been known to miss as much as one day of school per week due to pain and nausea, and many are home-schooled for this reason. The full range of costs associated with pediatric GERD have not been studied, nor have the costs associated with lack of treatment."

This disease is serious. Treat it with respect and stop shrugging it off, as a little spit up that will go away in a couple months. "GERD," as my mom said to me, "should be a household word," and I want the next person who comes to my door raising money for a cure to be trying to raise money for GERD.

CHAPTER NINE

SO YOU ASK: HOW'S SHE DOING?

Shae-Lynne is doing well. She has been doing better the past few months than she has since birth. Yet, I feel a sense of sadness. Everyone I see or talk to that asks how Shae-Lynne is doing, I am sure they expect the usual reply, "oh good," but I can never bring myself to say that. Now that she is doing well, I answer, "She is having a few *good* weeks," as I never know how long it will last.

I have been able to get Shae-Lynne's rate per hour (the amount pumped into her over an hour) up to seventy mls (almost 2.5 ozs); the highest it has ever been. This pleases me greatly as we are now able to unhook her for a couple of hours a day. Those few hours are the best of her day. She feels wonderful with no gagging at all. The rest of the day she gags from time to time and may have one or more vomits. This has come to be acceptable to me, and what I consider to be doing well. When I answer the question "How is she doing?" with *good*, I invariably hear, "Well, maybe she's finally outgrowing it."

It is now eleven p.m. I hooked Shae-Lynne up to her feeds shortly after nine and put her into bed. She just woke for the first time of the night (there will be many more) crying. She wakes gagging, crying, clawing at her throat, neck and chest. She rubs her eyes in exhaustion and her nose as though to rub it away. She gags again. As she continues to rub her nose, I wonder if it is also burning from reflux. After all, the vomit has come out of her nose before. Perhaps it is coming up into it now and not coming out. I hope this is not the case as I can imagine the damage gastric acid can do to her sinuses.

Good is such a relative word. Yes, she is doing good, but only compared to how she was doing. Every night we go through this around midnight (sometimes earlier), the gagging and pain. She is uncomfortable to say the very least and it wakes her. She is tired and tries desperately, through the gags and pain, to close her eyes and go back to sleep. She stirs, wiggles around and cries out in pain again. Her eyes open only momentarily to make sure Mommy is still there. I sing and hold Shae-Lynne trying to comfort her. If only she would throw up and get it over with, she could sleep. She begins to settle only before crying out in pain. I feel guilty because I am so sick of this. I find myself frustrated and angry. I try to remember that she cannot help herself. As her little body is heaving and choking I think it is easier to be angry than to think about how this must feel for her. I gently lift Shae-Lynne's hair out of her eyes and kiss the top of her head while holding her in my lap with the towel in front of her. I'm humming in her ear but don't think she can even hear me over the cries and high-pitched screams. Finally, she appears to be finished, three towels later. It is now well after midnight. Shae-Lynne finally falls asleep and I lay awake wondering if she is going to start again once I am comfortable.

At 2:53 a.m. Shae-Lynne is squirming and whining. *Oh no, not again*, I think. I roll over and take her into my arms. We lay together for another half hour while she whimpers and tries several times to vomit. Nothing comes up and eventually she dozes off again.

5:12 a.m., here we go again. Shae-Lynne gags over and over again, whimpering with an occasional cry for fifteen minutes to half an hour before dozing off again. First thing in the morning is her worst time of day. She will repeat this scene every twenty minutes or so for the next three hours before falling asleep for one or two more hours.

Good, by her standards, maybe. Good by anyone else's standards, I don't think so. Would I be feeling good, even with an empty stomach, if I felt what she felt every night and morning? No. You cannot explain all this when someone asks a simple question. So when I answer, *good*, I bite my tongue when I hear the inevitable, "She must be growing out of it then." Never mind that Shae-Lynne is now six months older than the age when we were told she was supposed to be when she would outgrow this disease. Yes, Shae-Lynne is doing very well indeed.

MY GIFT

By Alice Porembski
Merrimack, NH

I am a stranger to you now, but let me walk with you for awhile...
Because I have been where you are, and where you are about to go.
I have no answers.
I offer instead my hand, my heart, my listening ear, my time, and my experience....
So that one day you can turn to another and say:
I am a stranger to you now, but let me walk with you for awhile...
Because I have been where you are, and where you are about to go.
I have no answers.
I offer instead my hand, my heart, my listening ear, my time, and my experience....
So, that one day you can turn to another and say:

CHAPTER TEN

OTHERS SHARE THEIR STORIES

There are so many other families experiencing what Michael, Shae-Lynne and I have been living for the past few years. We want to share some of their stories. All of these stories are true and written in their own words. They too have found no answers.

First, we'll start with Melissa. Her story is long, as she has four children. All have suffered to some degree. Her youngest is Alyssa, now eight.

Melissa's Children

It's hard to put into words the frustration, pain and just not understanding this disease called GERD. I have four children. Justin was my first, born on February 1, 1982. When he was born, I was only sixteen. Being a young mother, I thought his constant projectile vomiting to be normal. Every feeding ended with a complete change of clothing for both he and I.

When Justin was just two weeks old his pediatrician changed formulas. Although I questioned the expiration date on the formula he had given me (October 1981), I was assured it would be good for six more months. Unfortunately, I listened to him. Now, along with the vomiting, my son had developed salmonella. He was treated and thankfully got recovered from the salmonella. The vomiting continued; however, the doctor was not concerned as Justin continued to gain weight. No tests were performed and he eventually stopped vomiting when he started solid foods.

My second child, Jeremy, now seventeen, never experienced the vomiting. However, he was hospitalized at five months with asthmatic bronchitis, but was not officially diagnosed with asthma until he turned seven. We went through the changing of medications, doctors, specialists, pulmonary clinics, allergy testing, breathing machines. We dealt with endless days of worrying when an asthma attack would occur. Nothing stops this child from succeeding in the goals he has planned for his life. At twelve he won first place in the county in high jump. He was also a runner. At fourteen he was erecting his own building. He made birdhouses and landscaped our property. He had complained of heartburn starting when he was twelve. He was prescribed Zantac and it seemed to help.

On July 5, 1999, the worst day of my life, we had just finished lunch. Jeremy said, "Mom, I can't swallow." I suggested he try his inhaler. The inhaler did not help. He was getting worse. He couldn't swallow or breathe. We headed to a nearby hospital by car. On the way I feared this was the last day of my child's life. It was a horrible feeling. He felt weak as though he may pass out, as he was still unable to breathe or swallow. At the emergency room, Jeremy was given a shot of Benedryl. They treated him for an allergic reaction and sent us home. He slept the rest of the afternoon. When he finally awoke he was still unable to swallow. This time I called the ambulance. I was not taking him back to the same hospital and I knew I could not get him to the hospital in the next town quickly enough. The EMTs, who were wonderful, thought he was experiencing spasm of the throat. Finally, after hours and hours of fear we were told it was "acid reflux." It was suggested that Jeremy see a specialist. By the time we were able to book an appointment, Jeremy had lost eleven pounds in five days. He could not eat anything except for cream of chicken soup through a straw. The specialist now put him on Carafate. It helped some. However, it was still quite awhile before he was able to do the endoscopy and give the official diagnoses of GERD. Jeremy was now prescribed Prevacid. It helped tremendously.

Recently a new symptom developed. Jeremy started coughing up excessive amounts of phlegm. By excessive I mean one hundred or more times a day. Thick, thick stuff that when he would cough, it would just fly out of his mouth or he would have to cough and cough to get it up because it was choking him. At the age of fourteen Jeremy had to leave school because of his health and be home-schooled. It was extremely embarrassing. The other kids asked why he always hacked like that. We changed doctors and then the numerous tests escalated. I lost count. We still have no answer as to why this continues. It is down to approximately fifty times per day.

My third child Joshua, now ten, was also a projectile vomitor, along with being labeled failure to thrive. At eight months, at our local hospital, Joshua had a barium x-ray, which showed Pyloric Stenosis. He was scheduled for surgery at Riley Hospital in Indianapolis, Indiana. Within twenty minutes the doctor from Riley informed us that there was nothing wrong with Joshua. The doctor felt our local hospital had not given Joshua enough barium to fully extend his stomach, thus the incorrect diagnosis. He continued to vomit until he was off the bottle. He is still very small for his age and is not a good eater.

My fourth child, Alyssa, is eight. She started from birth getting strangled on juice and water. She would choke and cry every time she was given the water or juice. She was a breast-fed baby as well as Joshua. Alyssa was sent to Riley Hospital for tests and as we watched on the monitor we could see the liquid go down into her windpipe. She was diagnosed with Esophageal Reflux. I was told she would "outgrow it" by the age of two. If she had not grown out of it by then, they would have to do surgery to correct the "flap" as they called it. Well she has not outgrown it. She was also choking on her own saliva usually when she was talking or running. I questioned a new doctor at the clinic about this problem. I thought he was very callous and he made me feel as though I was making too much of nothing, but he did order another barium swallow. Alyssa, now six, refused to drink much of the barium. The doctor said what little bit of barium we got in her did not show anything. When we returned to the "callous" doctor, he had the attitude like, "I told you so." Alyssa continues to be strangled by liquids at times. I'm still waiting for her to "outgrow" it.

No one can really understand the frustration of this disease unless you have gone through it yourself with your child. Mealtimes are supposed to be a good thing. But at every meal at our house, every noise we hear, we look to see if one of our children is choking. It is a constant worry. There has to be an answer. I know the answer for now is to never give up hope, love your children with all you have, and pray to God for a cure.

Melissa Payne, Boonville, Indiana

Next, we have Weru's story. Weru is a young boy from Africa. His mom, Lucy, had first contacted me by way of Shae-Lynne's web site. Weru, at the age of six months, had just been diagnosed with GERD and Lucy needed to learn more. We'll let her explain:

Lucy Tells Her Son Weru's Story

Weru, who is our second child, was born on 20th December 2000, at the Agha Khan Hospital, Nairobi. It was a difficult birth and very similar to his sister's, Wanjiku. As with Wanjiku's I arrived in hospital at 9:00 a.m. already dilated 4 cm but with no labor, by the time they were inducing labor I was already 7cm and still with no labor. It was only by the Grace of God that they did not vacuum him out when even with labor I could not sufficiently widen.

It was while still in hospital (I was there for three days and two nights) that something strange happened. On the second day (21st) at about 4:00 p.m., I had just finished breast-feeding the baby when suddenly he turned all red and started changing colour right in front of my eyes. I ran out in a panic and just before I reached the third bed there was a nurse; she grabbed the baby, turned him face downwards and started rubbing his back. I was watching the nurse and I realized that she was also scared. Just as suddenly as it had happened Weru was back to normal again as though nothing had ever been wrong. I remember the nurse asking me in Swahili (national language) whether I would just panic as I had if the baby choked when we got home.

Over the next few months Weru was okay and feeding just as well. Every so often (sometimes once a day or even thrice a day) the same thing that had happened would repeat itself and this occasionally caused some arguments between my husband and I because he claimed that I might not have burped the baby.

In May 2001, things took a turn for the worse. For almost two weeks we would have problems with him at night. He was not sleeping well and he seemed to have a fever that disappeared in the morning. We even took the baby to hospital and the doctor would not find anything wrong with him. On Saturday 9th of June 2001, Weru's temperature was so high that my husband and I decided to rush him to hospital, he was making funny voices. As soon as we got to the clinic we were rushed in to see the doctor, Weru's temperature was 41.8 high. We had to immediately rush him to Getrude's Garden Children's Hospital where we were admitted and after further investigation and a few X-rays it was discovered that Weru had pneumonia.

I would like to add that the week I spent in hospital was the most traumatic week, even now when I think about it I find that my eyes keep watering. I watched as every morning my baby was taken to some place where I was told that they removed mucus from his chest through whatever means they did. Weru would come back all red and crying and all this was so disturbing it always used to take me almost ten or so minutes to quiet him down.

We left for home after one week and everything seemed to be returning back to normal. After one week my daughter who is three developed a bad cough and my husband suggested that he would go back home at noon that day and take our daughter (she's asthmatic) to see the doctor. He arrived home at around 1:30 p.m. and instead of Wanjiku he found that Weru was running a temperature, which the nanny did not like. By the time he picked me up at 3:00 p.m., Weru was all wet and hot and mumbling. At the doctor's clinic, they immediately called an ambulance and we were rushed again to the children's hospital.

When Dr. Mbuthia came to see us that evening he felt that Weru's problem was not what we had initially thought, pneumonia again. According to him it was not possible to develop the same thing in less than a week. He felt that we needed to find out the root cause of the problem but for the night since Weru was having difficulty breathing he was put on oxygen. The next morning Weru was taken in for an endoscopy and this is when we discovered that he was suffering from reflux. In Weru's case, one of the stomach sphincters was weak or loose (not sure) but what happened was that after eating or drinking, the food/drink would then be brought up again. By this time some of it would be part acidic and this tended to erode his throat. We were then given Mucaine (antiacid), which was to be taken fifteen minutes before any meal. He was also put on Kiddi Phamarton (multivitamin), which would assist with his appetite among other things. We were also advised to prop him up after every meal and also whenever we put him to sleep.

From all this I have learned many things some painful and some wonderful. It has also taught my family a lot, in the case of my mother she had indicated that I might not have been keeping my children as warm as I should but after the diagnosis she was very understanding and helpful. My husband and I have learned to support each other a lot.

Lucy Mwangi
Kenya, Africa

I think Lucy's story shows how widespread infant GERD is. She also comments on the misunderstandings it created within her family. Trying her best and yet because Weru was not properly diagnosed, she was to blame. Again, I like her story as it shows there is hope and some do "grow out of it early."

After reading Weru's story I had a few questions for Lucy. This is how she answered them:

Questions

Q: How is Weru doing now?

Answer: He's progressed very well. The doctor will perform an edoscopy to see how far he's come.

Q: Did he vomit much?

A: Occasionally, mostly he was a silent refluxer, which explains why we took so long to discover and kept treating for other things.

Q: Did those medications help?

A: No, not immediately. We started seeing the change gradually after three months.

Q: Were you able to find enough help/support to make things easier?

A: Definitely, no! Nobody understands anything when I start talking about GERD or reflux. They could be Greek words as far as they are concerned. I was assisted by the Internet and through your daughter's story. It gave me courage; even though my son was not affected as Shae-Lynne at least he was not alone.

I remember that I came across Shae-Lynne's story the first time I surfed on the Internet looking for information on reflux. I cried as I read about her and when I got home I just held Weru and prayed for him and all other children who were going through so much pain at this early stage in life.

Lucy

Julie's story is especially heart wrenching as you read how Jared almost died.

Julie Shares Her Story about Jared

My second child, Jared, was a preemie born at thirty weeks gestation and spent eight weeks in the NICU. Before even coming home we noticed how often he would spit up his formula, but the nurses kept reassuring us this was very common and normal. Our older son had reflux when he was a baby, often spitting up an entire feeding right after he had taken a bottle. It never affected his desire or ability to eat, and it was really just a nuisance that he finally outgrew at fifteen months. When we saw Jared spitting up, we kept saying, "Oh no, we hope he doesn't develop reflux to the extent Jake had it." If only we had known how severe reflux could get, we would have been praying that his reflux was exactly like Jake's had been.

Toward the end of his stay in the NICU, everyone noticed that Jared was arching backward a lot, especially with feedings. Because this is often a sign of reflux, he had a scan done, which confirmed he was refluxing. We were told that, like our older son, this was something he would outgrow around the time he was a year old. He was placed on two medications for the reflux and shortly after was discharged home.

At home Jared was doing very well initially, although we had to be sure to elevate the head of his bassinette and keep him upright for at least a half hour after feedings because of the reflux. Then, one Sunday afternoon, just two weeks after he came home from the NICU, my husband was holding him while I got a bottle ready for his next feeding. Although his last feeding was over three hours earlier, he suddenly and unexpectedly vomited. The vomit came out his mouth and nose and he was unable to breathe. As my husband continued to hold him it suddenly became obvious Jared was unable to clear his airway and was choking. I grabbed a bulb syringe and tried sucking out his nose and mouth but was unable to clear him. He was quickly turning blue and I called 911 while my husband attempted CPR. In the few minutes it took for the ambulance to get to our house I changed from calm and focused to nearly hysterical as I looked at my blue, lifeless baby, unable to believe that after all we had gone through with him already, we were going to lose him like this. Just as the paramedics pulled up, Jared went completely limp and my husband was finally able to get a breath into him. He started to breathe and the paramedics gave him oxygen and took us to the hospital for our first of many hospital stays.

After the choking incident we were referred to see specialists at a children's hospital in our state. Jared's reflux medications were changed and we were sent home. Two weeks later he vomited and began choking again, so this time the specialist admitted us to the hospital for a few days. They changed his medications again, and this time he had no vomiting episodes while in the hospital. Everyone was pleased and ready to send us home. Before leaving, I pointed out to the doctor that the amount of his feedings he had gotten in the hospital was much less than normal and less than he needed, and that he had actually lost weight in the four days we were there. The doctor reassured us this was nothing to be concerned about and sent us home.

At home things continued to get worse. Jared would only take an ounce of formula and would refuse any more. What he did take he ended up vomiting anyway. We took him to our pediatrician and I cried as he was weighed and it showed he had lost more weight. The doctor put in an NG tube for feeding, telling us it would only be in a few weeks to build his weight back up.

With the NG tube in, Jared began refusing the bottle even more and his vomiting continued to get worse. We went back to the children's hospital, knowing that a G-tube was going to be recommended. When we met with the GI specialist he recommended both the G-tube and the Nissen fundoplication surgery. He sent the surgeon in to speak with us. Thankfully, the surgeon said he felt the Nissen was not appropriate at that time and we scheduled surgery for the G-tube only.

In hindsight it seems ridiculous that even the G-tube was recommended. Here we were putting feedings directly into Jared's stomach, which he would just vomit up anyway. He consequently developed a severe oral aversion from associating eating with pain and vomiting and completely stopped eating orally. After six months of poor weight gain, Jared had a week where he literally threw up every single feeding. I called the GI specialist who said the only option left was the Nissen. We decided to see our pediatrician, who agreed to send us to the other children's hospital in our state, for another opinion. When the new GI specialist came in to see Jared, he immediately said Jared's problem was a motility disorder of his stomach and that he needed a GJ feeding tube to give him feedings into his intestines, bypassing the stomach. The next morning they put in the tube. After only gaining eight in the two months, Jared suddenly began gaining an ounce a day with the new tube. While we were so happy to finally have an option that allowed Jared to gain weight, we were kicking ourselves for staying with the first hospital and GI specialist for so long. The new specialist also said the Nissen was inappropriate for children with motility disorders. We thank God we got a second opinion before going through with a surgery that was not only unnecessary but would have made him even worse.

After a few months we changed the GJ tube to a more permanent J-tube. While Jared continues to have excellent weight gain, he still continues to vomit throughout the day and night. It's almost unbelievable this is possible, as the only thing in his stomach is a small amount of gastric juice. He takes no nutrition orally. We're thrilled to see him thriving, but it is very difficult to watch him heaving and in so much discomfort because of the underlying motility disorder.

Unfortunately there are no effective treatments at this time. We've been told this is a condition he most likely will not outgrow, so we hope and pray that new treatments are developed in the future so that someday he can learn to eat again and get through life without vomiting every day. In the meantime, it helps to meet other people going through the same thing to share ideas and experiences, and just to feel we are not alone in dealing with a condition that can feel so isolating.

Julie Paschke
Appleton, WI

Sonia explains how two of her three girls were affected by GERD. It is so sad that Tasha, her oldest, had gone so long before being diagnosed.

Sonia Tells about Her Daughters

I have three daughters. Tasha is my oldest. She is fifteen and has GERD. Brittney, my middle child, has never had any stomach problems. She is now thirteen. The youngest, Sydnie, has GERD.

Tasha was sick as a baby. I was told she had colic. When she continued to have stomach problems I asked if colic could last that long. She was put through so many tests that were not even related to reflux. I just wanted someone to find out why my child acted the way she did. People teased me and said that I didn't feed her. Not one person understood. I didn't even understand. One doctor told me she was spoiled, one said she had asthma, and another said allergies were to blame. I took Tasha to the emergency room many times for stomach pain and endless crying. Tasha really didn't take much of a bottle. She took small amounts and spit up. I put her on baby food early thinking anything to satisfy her. She was sick a lot. She was eleven years old before diagnosed with GERD. A doctor in the emergency room discovered it. Tasha was eating roast and began to choke. She could breathe, but was having severe pain in her chest. I rushed her to the ER. An x-ray revealed that something was lodged in her throat. After finally getting the very small piece of meat out of her throat the ER doctor asked if Tasha had reflux. Tasha was referred to a specialist for an upper GI. The esophagus was so narrow that everything would get stuck. The specialist immediately did a scope and that was the big find. She had so much damage to her esophagus. She was put on Pepsid and that didn't help. The doctor finally put her on Prevacid. Tasha seemed to be better. She had to have another scope and it was decided that the dose was to be increased. She was taking sixty mgs. daily— thirty in the a.m. and thirty in the p.m. She started having breathing trouble and began choking again. Another scope revealed strictures. Tasha's esophagus was so damaged that the reflux had to be stopped. The doctor asked how I felt about a fundoplication. I said no. Then I was informed that with the surgery maybe it wouldn't turn into cancer. Without surgery— almost positive she would get cancer before she was thirty. I decided to have the fundo.

I was three months pregnant with my youngest child when Tasha had the surgery. She had a tough time for several days. We were in the hospital for six days. That was a year ago August 4th. I asked Tasha the other day if she was glad we had the surgery and she said yes. She would do it all over again if she had to. She told me that the pain in her chest and throat was terrible and she never wanted to have it again. She loves that she can eat meat and other foods. She still has to stay away from carbonated drinks, as she can't burp or throw up. That is bad when she gets a stomach bug or has a drink that is carbonated. She still feels it is much better than the way she was before. She had to have her esophagus stretched a few months ago. She may have to have that done every three to six months.

My eleven-month-old has had a time with GERD also. Sydnie was diagnosed three weeks old. I am hoping that it was caught early enough so that her esophagus will not be damaged. Sydnie takes Prevacid. She was first put on Reglan and Zantac. The Reglan made her head shake and her arms tremor. She still projectile vomits. When she was put on Prevacid I could tell the difference right away. She is doing well now. It has certainly been a roller coaster ride, so I don't want to get my hopes up. Now she is improving and has gained weight. It is nice not to have to take towels and ten outfits and fifty bibs every time I leave the house. I just hope she continues to improve.

I don't know if anything I have told you will help. I sure hope that other children will not have to suffer as my oldest child did because no one could diagnose her and no medicine was given for eleven years. I know that doctors are more aware now than they were then. I just hope they continue to learn more and help these children. God bless you. Thank you for caring.

> Sonia Lee
> Ringgold, Georgia

Next, we have Patti telling her son's story. Keep in mind these are real people telling *their* child's/children's story. They are real. Although Spencer seems to have had reflux worse than anyone could imagine. It is nonetheless true—this does happen.

I am awed by the attitudes of both Patti and Spencer. To have endured what they have and for the length of time they have, it is incredible that they both remain so positive.

Patti with Spencer's Story

Spencer was born on Valentine's Day, 1989. His entry into this world was far from how I had anticipated. Instead of having a quiet peaceful birth, it was surrounded by all kinds of medical technology. Spencer had to be suctioned to avoid aspirating meconium. He was then taken to a warmer bed to be suctioned more. Being in distress led to him being taken to NICU where he spent the next three weeks recovering from an infection in his blood called sepsis.

At feeding time, Spencer had a difficult time taking formula and would spit up frequently. He was diagnosed with gastro esophageal reflux. I didn't know much about it but thought it wasn't too big of a deal as all babies spit up.

Within ten days, I learned otherwise. Spencer refluxed and aspirated during a night feeding. He also stopped breathing and turned blue. This time, at the hospital, he was diagnosed with aspiration pneumonia. He recovered well and came home. At home, I continued to do all that I knew. Every time he spit up, I re-fed what he spit up. Most of my day revolved around feeding Spencer. Fortunately, there weren't any more episodes to scare me as that had.

We were so happy when Spencer was about one; I noticed he stopped spitting up. I thought that things were finally settling down. He had frequent ear infections and other respiratory infections but I didn't think much about that nor did the pediatrician. As time went on, he started having symptoms that should have made all of us think more. He started wheezing and coughing at night. I would go into his room and find him blue. I continually brought him to the ER and to the pediatrician but when he was there he was fine so they didn't do anything. The doctor I worked for finally convinced Spencer's pediatrician that there was something wrong that forced me to sleep sitting upright so Spencer could lean against me, as he couldn't sleep lying down. We then began home monitoring with an apnea monitor and pulse oximeter.

The apnea monitor showed frequent oxygen desaturation. Oxygen saturation should be at or above 95%. Spencer frequently dropped into the 60s and 70s. He was then being treated for asthma but that wasn't helping the problems at night.

It did not help when at age two Spencer's adenoids were removed, hoping to help his respiratory problems. When he was three his tonsils were removed, which did not help. We then saw a pulmonologist as his respiratory problems continued. Immediately, the pulmonologist suspected reflux as being Spencer's problem despite the fact that he didn't spit up. His suspicions were confirmed when we saw a pediatric gastroenterologist. A pH probe done revealed Spencer was refluxing 25% of the time. He was started on medication. An endoscopy was done which showed that he also had esophagitis due to long-term refluxing of acid. We tried different med combinations. We tried changing the meds and raising the doses. Nothing worked. Spencer was losing weight. He was miserable. All he would eat was yogurt.

I changed GI doctors and although the meds were almost doubled, things did not improve. Three more endoscopies performed showed worsening esophagitis. It was now decided that due to the degree of esophagitis, as well as Spencer's ongoing respiratory problems, surgery was the best choice at this time.

Determined and relieved that this was indeed the answer for my son, now almost four years old, off we went to the surgeon's. He explained that they would make an incision and take the top portion of the stomach and wrap it around the esophagus to tighten the sphincter muscle that wasn't functioning and was allowing the reflux. This surgery, which is called a Nissen fundoplication, was done. Recovery was hard. When it was time for Spencer to eat, he drank and vomited. He ate and vomited. This went on for several days. We couldn't take him off IV fluids because he couldn't get anything down. Two weeks after surgery, the surgeon decided to do an upper GI to check things out. It was found that the "wrap" was too tight. Spencer only had a 1 mm opening for things to go through. It was barely adequate for saliva. The next morning, Spencer went back to the OR to have his wrap dilated. Almost immediately afterward he could eat. No problems at all.

As time went by, it was obvious that not only could Spencer eat, he could reflux too. It was very upsetting to watch this happen. The symptoms weren't as bad as they had been but things weren't pleasant. I took Spencer back to the doctor many times. The doctor felt Spencer was not refluxing because the fundoplication had been performed.

The pH probe and endoscopy were repeated and the results showed that he was indeed refluxing again. I think the doctors really took things to heart when Spencer had a GI bleed in December, which was only eleven months after surgery. At only four years old, Spencer came into my room at 5:00 a.m. to tell me that he was burping up blood. My poor baby! All we went through to have the initial surgery done and here he was worse yet.

Just ten days short of a year after Spencer's first abdominal surgery, he had his second abdominal surgery. This time it was an uncut Collis-Nissen fundoplication performed by a different surgeon. He also had a pyloroplasty done to aid with stomach emptying. This surgery was longer and more difficult than the first. However, after he recovered, it seemed like the surgery was helping. Eating was difficult again but there was no anatomic reason.

Things were progressing nicely until about nine months after surgery when Spencer started having painful episodes of vomiting. This was very unusual and very different from anything I had ever seen with him. We went back to the GI. After another endoscopy was performed, the doctor told me there was a second hole from the stomach to the esophagus, which allowed Spencer to reflux. There was a lot of inflammation around it since acid probably just sat there all the time. This needed to be corrected.

We went back to the same surgeon who had done the second surgery and Spencer had his third abdominal surgery in less than two years! Because Spencer was losing weight, the doctor placed a feeding tube. Recovery was a little bit easier this time thanks to the feeding tube. We didn't have to worry about Spencer's eating as much. However, even with the G-tube, Spencer didn't gain weight well. At six years old, he only weighed thirty-six pounds.

Spencer had several severe infections of the G-tube site during the first several months and was hospitalized three times for cellulites and once for a necrotic abscess and peritonitis (thanks to a little boy who pulled his tube partially out). The doctor did an endoscopy while in the hospital about five months after the third surgery and found that Spencer still had esophagitis. This meant the third surgery hadn't worked at all.

We then spent the next two years trying to figure out why fundoplications weren't successful for Spencer. We were told that the success rate is typically >90%. Why didn't Spencer fall into this category? We tried high dose steroids to see if it made any difference in his oral intake and then repeated an endoscopy to see if there was inflammation present while on steroids. There was. We also tried an elimination diet. Spencer had a couple of foods that we knew he wasn't allergic to and was able to eat them. Otherwise, all he had was a formula called Neocate 1+ through his G-tube. We did this for several weeks and repeated the endoscopy. Unfortunately, still no improvement.

Spencer needed the best. I felt Boston Children's Hospital was the place to go and took Spencer there in June 1997. In a whirlwind week, Spencer had the full scope of GI testing done. He had lab work, an upper GI, pH probe, esophageal manometry, and an endoscopy. They found that his previous fundoplication was completely disrupted. His esophageal sphincter muscle was so far open the doctor could see out Spencer's mouth with the scope while in the stomach. There continued to be reflux, esophagitis, and esophageal dysmotility. The GI doctor there suggested that we try medications for the dysmotility first in addition to the reflux meds he was already taking. We tried one medication—it helped the dysmotility but made the horrible reflux worse. Another was tried with the same effect. When those medications failed, it was again time to consider surgery.

Spencer had his fourth abdominal surgery done by a surgeon at Boston Children's Hospital. This surgeon was kind, caring and explained the possible procedures he was planning. He wouldn't know just what he would do until he was in the OR. After twelve hours in the OR, Spencer went to the

ICU after having a partial esophagogastrectomy, new gastrostomy, and modified Belsey fundoplication. Recovery was more difficult than any of the other surgeries and perhaps harder than all three combined. However, the surgery was successful. After several months, Spencer was weaned from G-tube feedings and was doing well. The G-tube was removed ten months after surgery. Spencer was medication free and we were thrilled!

He started to experience some abdominal pain, diarrhea and dizziness about fifteen months after the fourth surgery. He had episodes of dizziness in the past as well, which we could never find a reason for. It was determined by the GI doctor in Boston that Spencer had dumping syndrome. This is when the stomach is emptying too rapidly. It happens frequently when the stomach is small. By this point Spencer's was very small. We were able to easily treat it with diet and cornstarch, which helps to control blood sugar. Things were good again. Spencer went to summer camp for the first time and loved it! He stayed four weeks.

After camp, however, he was burping and hiccupping which were always signs of reflux for him. We called the GI doctor and started Zantac. That didn't help so he started Prilosec. Testing was done yet again. The pH probe showed that despite not eating for most of the test, Spencer was indeed refluxing and there was mild esophagitis. The doctor added medications. Things were under control for a while and summer came. Spencer went back to camp for a total of eight weeks! I went to see him after two weeks. He looked horrible. Dark circles, hoarseness, coughing, and most of all, he didn't want to eat even though we were taking him out for some fast food!

I talked to the GI doctor who felt that it was probably time to consider surgery. I thought and thought and thought some more. It just sounded so complicated. Much more complicated than any of the prior surgeries. I consulted with surgeons all around the country. There was one in LA, one in Salt Lake City, the surgeon who did Spencer's fourth surgery was in Madison, WI, and we also consulted a very seasoned surgeon in Boston.

The surgeon in LA wanted to remove Spencer's stomach and attach it to his small intestine. The surgeon in Salt Lake City wanted to replace his esophagus with colon. The surgeon in Madison wanted to replace the bottom portion of his esophagus with small intestine since the small intestine has motility, which would push anything that Spencer refluxed back into his stomach. However, he would only do it if the surgeon who trained him flew out to help. The surgeon who trained him was the surgeon in Boston. The doctor in Madison suggested that we go straight to Boston, as it would be better for Spencer to be in Boston.

Shortly after Labor Day 2000, we went to visit Hardy Hendren, MD, at Boston Children's Hospital. We had spoken in early August so he was familiar with the case. He suggested the same surgery that his former protégée in Madison had suggested. Obviously that was going to be the procedure we would pursue. He also felt that he might take part of Spencer's colon to enlarge his stomach, as his stomach was "tiny." Dr. Hendren is a very busy man even though he is much older than your average pediatric surgeon at age seventy. The first open day he had in the OR was December 13, 2000. Spencer was scheduled.

Early in the morning on December 13th, Spencer's prep for the surgery ended. It had started more than twelve hours earlier. At about 7:30 a.m. Spencer, his father, and I went to the OR. Spencer went into the OR at about 8:00 a.m. Dr. Hendren came to talk with us. He writes his own consent forms so that nothing is ever left out. After that, Spencer was in Dr. Hendren's hands. He remained there for almost sixteen hours. At about midnight, Dr. Hendren emerged from the OR and immediately told me we had done the right thing as our GI doctor had changed his mind and hadn't been in agreement. Spencer's esophagus had been "destroyed." He wasn't able to do the stomach as he felt he'd already been there too long. I agreed. Obviously, this recovery was far more difficult. Spencer had problems with pleural effusions, pneumonia, a leak at the atastamosis where the esophagus and small intestine were joined, and a GI bleed. He remained in the ICU for about a week and was on a ventilator for the first three days. He continued to require oxygen for about two weeks. Things finally improved and he went home on G-tube feedings at the end of January.

By February, Spencer told me he was refluxing a LOT. Back to the hospital we went where Spencer stayed for another two weeks. It was then decided that Spencer definitely needed surgery to enlarge his stomach. At home again, things weren't good. Spencer was losing weight so we went back again to have a new kind of feeding tube placed that although you could feed into the stomach it also had a port that bypassed the stomach. It took about two weeks to increase his feedings but once there, he gained weight like crazy! Twenty-five pounds in three months! Spencer went back to school in mid April. He managed to pass all of his advanced sixth grade classes and was allowed to progress to all seventh grade advanced classes!

In late July, after being able to enjoy several baseball games, a trip to the Jersey shore, and a trip to Fredericksburg, Virginia, we headed back to

Boston to have the gastric augmentation. I wasn't feeling very good about things. I had no clue if the surgery would work or not but I knew that Spencer couldn't stay on his J-tube feedings forever. So, another huge surgery prep began. Spencer went into the OR this time at about 11:00 a.m. and was out by midnight. His surgical recovery was smooth this time! He and I were very excited! However, when it was time to start feeding, it didn't go well. Spencer wasn't hungry and wouldn't take anything orally. They tried his G-tube at a low rate. However, what was left after three hours of feeding was more than what had gone in! With medications added and time, things got good enough that Spencer could be fed and we could go home!

Remarkably, Spencer was able to start school on time and is doing well enough to be on the honor roll! He even got a B+ in Algebra! He continues to have problems with gastric emptying but is now on a new medication, which is helping much more than anything else has. He continues to require tube feedings but happily eats orally as well and almost never forgets to ask for lunch money in the morning!

We have traveled a long, bumpy road and I'm sure we aren't at the end. Spencer's experiences in life appear to be shaping his future. He has very high goals set. He wants to be just like his surgeon! Dr. Hendren told him that he could do better than that! Spencer certainly has the potential to be a pediatric surgeon. He's a very bright and assertive young man. However, I tell him that as long as he's a happy and productive human being, I will be more than proud! I sing Dr. Hendren's praises wherever I go. I can't even begin to think about where Spencer would be today without Dr. Hendren.

Patti
Pittsburgh, PA

The Reason For This Book

The following are a few messages left in the guest book on Shae-Lynne's website:

I have a twenty-one-month-old with FTT and sensory dysfunction. We have a feeding tube in her nose now for two weeks and go in the hospital Tuesday for a G-tube and Nissen Fundoplication surgery. We are so scared for her. Grace does not want to eat. We have been battling this since birth. At twenty-one months Grace is seventeen pounds. I understand how you feel and would love to talk further with you.

* * *

I have read about your story and I can relate to a lot of your heartaches. We have a three-month-old boy who was diagnosed with GERD. He currently is taking Zantac and Metoclopramide. Fortunately he is weighing in at nineteen pounds (way above normal weight). We obviously don't have a thriving problem…. But he only nurses for about five minutes every four to five hours because it is so difficult for him to eat. He gags and chokes throughout the whole feeding. (I'm sure genetics play a key role with his size.)

But all throughout the day he has difficultly breathing! He is gagging and coughing all the time. I dread the nighttime because he struggles to sleep with his breathing problems. They say that it is common with GERD but it only seems to be getting worse. I use the humidifier…prop him up…use the saline drops and nothing seems to work. Have you heard of anyone else with these types of problems? I just started doing some research on my own and I first stumbled onto your site.

Thank you for sharing your story and your information. It helps mothers like me know that I'm not the only one who feels there has to be some other ways of helping these children. Hope to hear from you soon.

* * *

My daughter is seven months old and barely weighs thirteen pounds. I don't know if it's GERD yet, as of now she is on medication for reflux. It's still too soon to tell if it's working. It's only been four days. Should I see a difference immediately with the meds, or am I another paranoid mother? She's so tiny, and it breaks my heart to think that she's not getting what she needs as far as nourishment. Is there anything else I can do to ease this? I'm so glad I'm not the only one going through this. Thank goodness!

* * *

Unfortunately, both of our boys are GERD kiddos. David is now three years old; Caleb is nine months. While David didn't require (fundo), Caleb did due to breathing complications. At any rate I was curious as to whether there is an online support system/list/e-group for parents w/GERD babies? Thanks.

* * *

Our thoughts and prayers are with you. You have a wonderful, brave little girl. Our journey with this is just beginning with our son, and your story is inspiration to us—thank you so much for sharing.

* * *

I just read about your little one and can certainly relate! It is so unfair what our children go through.... My son has suffered so much and has had the Nissen Fundoplication, the first one at five and one half weeks of age; he is now three and one-half years and still suffers.

* * *

Thank you for sharing your story. I have an eight-week-old nephew who was just recently diagnosed with reflux. He has already been hospitalized twice already for it and is now on Zantac to see if it would help him. He weighs 8 lbs. 12 oz. and is still gaining good though as he was born weighing 4 lbs. 12 oz. Your story has helped my sister realize that she isn't the only one going through this. Thank you very much.

* * *

Hi, your site made me feel so much better as my little girl Stacie who is nine and one half months old and weighing 14 lbs, 5 ounces (birth 7 lbs. 13 oz.) was diagnosed with reflux at three months. She refused feed in the hospital, failure to thrive, and all sorts of tests, N/G tube now, and looking at having a G-tube put in as still not eating. Waiting for MRI in June for any sign of neurological problem. Has large head 95-100th percentile for age. Has a dietician, OT since release from sick kids hospital under the care of pediatric GI specialist and feeding team. Vomits less now that is on Prilosec...my husband and I were curious about Shae-Lynne's progress. I also needed to let you know that all your hard work on your web site meant a lot to me, as I truly know how little time you had. Thanks.

* * *

My daughter is six years old and has a bad case of GERD. I know what you are going thru. We vomit all the time and never a day goes by without a bellyache. I wish more research could be done also for children with GERD! Even if it is uncommon. Prayers to God, we should lift this up to God daily! God can do anything!

* * *

I am searching for the cause/solution to my son's vomiting and retching. At three and one half years old we have dealt with the vomiting since he was eight months old and developed hydrocephalus. He was born with a brain malformation and has a shunt but the vomiting is considered unrelated. At fifteen months, he weighs less than thirteen pounds and was so severely dehydrated that his life was in danger and we had a G-tube placed. The vomiting continued and so a J-tube was placed through the G-tube to try feeding by bypassing the stomach. He managed to throw the tube up out of his intestine, back into the stomach and up this throat where he choked on it. He ended up in a trauma emergency room for that episode. So in January 2001, we had a J-tube surgically placed. The vomiting and retching continues. It can be just thick mucous, yellow/green bile, formula or any combination. It occurs day and night, awake or asleep and the Zantac and Reglan are doing nothing. I understand your frustration and fears as I share the same ones. Here's to a mom who keeps searching for help for our children.

* * *

I was looking for information on reflux as my son has had it since he was born and your website caught my eye. What a beautiful tribute to your daughter as well as your mother. I'm speechless and in tears. God bless you all. My prayers go out to you.

* * *

I'm very sorry to hear about your daughter's condition but I know that God has a way of dealing with everything. I'm sure that she will grow out of it. I do want to commend you for taking action and making people aware of this rare condition. I know that other parents are happy to know that they're not alone in this situation. I'll be praying for you and your daughter. God bless.

* * *

My daughter Payton is nine weeks old. She too has been diagnosed with severe GERD. She is on Zantac and Reglan and due to an apnea episode she is on a monitor for sleeping. We are told that she would hopefully outgrow this but you feel so helpless when you're going through it now. Thank God I have a great babysitter who has taken an interest in Payton's needs. She only watches my daughter and makes me feel confident in her abilities when I am at work. Secondly my daughter was born with a deviated left pupil. It is ever so slight. We have seen an ophthalmologist after staying on the pediatrician about a referral. The deviation is called corectopia. Her vision is intact and the eye doctor said that this might only be cosmetic. But still I could hardly handle one more thing. So I can empathize with you in the latest findings of Shae. She is a beautiful little girl…I pray that all heals well for her and thank you for this opportunity to talk to someone else who understands that GERD is more severe than what some say.

* * *

I have a son that has a genetic disorder. It is Partial Trisomy 17. He is now seven months old. We have dealt with reflux from the time of his birth. I can relate so much. He had a G-tube placed at the age of two weeks as well as a

Nissen and has slow gastric emptying. He is taking more by mouth now than tube. It doesn't seem to matter how he is fed. It still seems to come back up. He weighs seven pounds twelve ounces. He has the gagging spells that seem to last forever and you can tell they hurt and are very uncomfortable. The doctors seem to relate it to his disorder and state that there isn't much else we can do. I feel that if he could keep his feedings down that he would grow. I know how you feel, and feel free to e-mail me anytime. Thank you.

* * *

My daughter is very similar to yours. My Ally has suffered with GERD for almost two years now. I truly understand what you are going through. May God bless you and your daughter. You are doing a wonderful job with her care.

CHAPTER ELEVEN

MEDICINES/SURGERY

This book may detail Shae-Lynne's life thus far but it is not for her or about her. There are children all over the world living variations of this same story. These infants have one thing in common—constant pain. This book is for them. This is for their moms and dads who think they are alone and don't know where to turn. This is for the general public who (like me before Shae-Lynne) haven't even heard of GERD. This is for anyone who has been plagued with chronic heartburn and pops antacids like candy. This book has been written about a chronic disease for which there is no cure. Usually ignored and almost never taken seriously, GERD can cause many complications, severely affect a person's quality of life and even in some cases death.

In this chapter you will find information on GERD. We will also explain more completely some of the medications used to treat this disease. And finally, a little bit about fundoplication.

Gastro Esophageal Reflux Disease

Every person regardless of age or race has experienced reflux at some time or another, particularly after meals. Most people don't even realize it is happening. Some refer to this as heartburn. Actually heartburn is really just a symptom of what is happening.

Briefly, let me explain the way our digestive system is supposed to work.

The digestive system refers to everything from the mouth to the anus. The process of digestion begins in the mouth as we chew. The food is broken down, and is mixed with saliva (this begins the chemical action needed for digestion). Using our tongue the food gets forced to the back of our throat or pharynx. It then moves into the esophagus where muscles relax and contract in a rhythmic motion—called peristalsis—squeezing it down towards the stomach. The esophagus is found directly behind the trachea or windpipe. At the bottom of the esophagus a valve called the Lower Esophageal Sphincter (LES) opens to allow the food to pass into the stomach. When the LES is working properly it closes tightly to prevent the food from being pushed backwards up into the esophagus.

Once the food is in the stomach it is mixed with digestive juice made up of pepsin and hydrochloric acid. The food particles are further broken down before moving through the pyloric sphincter at the bottom of the stomach and into the small intestine. The small intestine consists of three parts: the duodenum, jejunum, and ileum. As food moves through these parts more digestive juices will be added to the mixture and the majority of our nutrients are absorbed.

From the third part of the small intestine (ileum) the leftovers are moved into the large intestine or colon where eighty to ninety percent of the water is absorbed and the waste moves through the anal canal and out the anus.

Obviously this is a very brief description of a hugely complex process but ideally this is how things should work. Many things can go wrong throughout this process; not the least of which is reflux. Reflux occurs when the LES fails to close properly or relaxes. This causes food and stomach juices (including the hydrochloric acid) to flow into the esophagus, and in some cases into the windpipe and lungs and out of the mouth and even nose. The stomach has a thick lining to protect itself from the acid that is produced; the esophagus and throat do not. The refluxed material can leave you with a bitter or sour taste in your mouth and/or a burning sensation behind the breastbone that many times has been mistaken for a heart attack as it can mimic those symptoms by radiating to the neck, throat and even arms. Sixty million Americans experience heartburn at least once a month as reported by The American College of Gastroenterology and more than ten percent suffer daily.

The United States Department of Health and Human Services, according to statistics, state that most of the time reflux is merely an occasional annoyance. However, more than seven million Americans do suffer from the more serious condition known as Gastro Esophageal Reflux Disease.

Complications

Reflux is referred to as GERD when it begins to cause complications and requires treatment. Many of the complications are very serious and even in some cases potentially fatal. Many of these are referred to as atypical, meaning they are not considered the norm; however, they occur in a major number of GERD cases.

IN INFANTS AND CHILDREN

Failure to Thrive—Constant vomiting of entire feedings can cause poor weight gain and even weight loss.

Food and Oral Aversions—Associations made between food and pain or unpleasantness can cause many infants to begin refusing food (as with Shae-Lynne). As a parent this is one of the more frustrating complications. Many times nothing short of tube feeding will provide the proper nutrition. Most people assume you are not approaching the situation properly or have not tried the right food. They assume that if the child gets hungry enough he/she will eat. Unfortunately, in too many cases this is untrue. The fear of pain that food brings is stronger than the desire/instinct to eat. I told a friend one day, "Shae-Lynne hasn't gotten to the point of a surgically inserted feeding tube because she refused her peas last night!" I was trying to get across it was after months of struggle and several doctors' opinions that the tube was inserted as a last resort. There is no doubt in my mind that Shae-Lynne would have starved herself to death if not for the feeding tube.

Vomiting—Definitely the messiest of the complications. This can be anything from the easy spit up that most people associate with babies to the heaving, retching, gagging and choking Shae-Lynne exhibits. As mentioned before, this can become so severe as to cause failure to thrive.

Gagging and/or Choking—Can be accompanied with vomiting, although some infants gag and choke when eating or throughout the day for no apparent reason.

Apnea—An episode in which the child stops breathing for more than ten to twenty seconds and can occur any time of the day or night. Infants who have frequent apnea episodes require an apnea monitor, especially through the night.

Aspiration Pneumonia—Aspiration is when food or refluxed material is allowed to enter the lungs. This causes breathing problems and in some causes recurrent pneumonias and respiratory problems.

Constant Inconsolable Crying—We all know how heartbreaking it can be when we are unable to help our infant cope with pain they are experiencing.

INFANTS AND ADULTS

Asthma—Studies show that up to 80 percent of people with asthma also have reflux. Now, scientists are beginning to believe that GERD may be the cause of asthma in certain cases. It's thought that when the refluxed material enters the airway and lungs it can cause bronchial spasms and long-term lung damage.

Barrett's Esophagus—The stomach is protected from its acid by specialized cells called columnar epithelium cells but the esophagus is not. This condition occurs when the more delicate esophageal cells called squamous epithelium are chronically burned and damaged. In an attempt at protecting against the acid, the body begins replacing these cells with a special type of columnar epithelium cells similar to those found in the stomach. It is unknown why but these new cells become pre-cancerous.

Cancer—Often the result of years of ignoring heartburn; the survival rate is low because symptoms usually only appear after it has progressed to other areas of the body, thus putting a diagnosis off until it's too late.

Chronic Cough, Hoarseness or Laryngitis—Caused by refluxed stomach acid damaging the throat and vocal cords. In some cases this may be the only symptom of GERD. See your doctor if you (or your baby) have a cough or hoarseness lasting three weeks or more.

Chronic Pain

Dysphagia—difficulty swallowing and strictures. The main cause of dysphagia is severe scarring in the esophagus from constant acid exposure. The scar tissue is thicker than the normal lining of the esophagus causing strictures that can, in effect, clog the esophagus and prevent food and even liquids from passing through.

Difficulty (or Noisy) Breathing

Esophageal Bleeding and Anemia—Caused by blood loss, anemia means your hemoglobin count (distributes oxygen to the body's cells and carries carbon dioxide back to the lungs) is lower than normal. Reflux can cause anemia by eating away at the esophagus until it begins to bleed.

Esophagitis—Inflammation of the esophagus caused by contact with stomach acid.

Eroded Dental Enamel—Stomach acid entering the mouth can erode the teeth. I am reminded of a story I read months back about a mother who continually took her son to the dentist because his teeth were as she called it disintegrating. For a couple of years the dentist blamed her for not making sure he brushed properly. Eventually she switched dentists and the new dentist recognized the damage and sent them to a GI. He was diagnosed with GERD and because he was a silent reflux (no symptoms), it had gone untreated for years and had progressed to Barrett's esophagus.

Frequent Burping or Hiccupping

Poor Sleep

Ulceration or Strictures in the Esophagus

Treatments

There are several ways to treat reflux/GERD that generally begins with lifestyle and dietary changes, progresses to medication and ultimately failing all that, surgery. In this section I will briefly explain each, where appropriate they relate to infants through adults.

If you are reading this to find some answers to problems experienced by you or your infant, I hope that you are in the majority and that something you read helps you. If you are in the minority and have tried everything listed below without success, I can only say you are not alone and my heart goes out to you.

Thickened Feeds—In some cases your infant's doctor may instruct you to add a small amount of cereal to the bottle. Never do this on your own. Consult your doctor before adding anything to your child's bottle. It sounds reasonable that thicker milk may be more likely to stay down. Unfortunately, if your infant is refusing food as Shae-Lynne was, this suggestion is slightly ridiculous. When we tried this with Shae-Lynne she took even less milk than usual and then threw up milk with cereal in it. Enfamil and/or Enfalac AR are infant formulas on the market made with added rice starch specifically for this purpose. The formula is only slightly thicker than regular formulas when mixed. As it reaches the stomach and mixes with stomach acid, it is supposed to thicken even more. Consult your pediatrician before trying this.

Positioning—Keep your child in an upright position during and after feeds. Raise the head of the bed/crib by at least six inches. I always kept four pillows under the head of Shae-Lynne's crib and placed rolled-up towels around each of her sides and under her bum to keep her from sliding down. This worked well until she got old enough to get up on her own. There are several wedges and sling type devices sold to get the same affect but I never bothered to spend the money on them since the rolled towels and sheets did the trick.

Dietary Manipulation—Many times in infants reflux is exacerbated by a milk protein allergy. In many cases switching to a hypoallergenic formula will help. Children and adults should remove foods and/or medications from their diet that make reflux worse. This includes chocolate, fats, caffeine, licorice, carbonated beverages, alcohol, nicotine, theophylline, beta agonists, calcium channel blockers, narcotics, benzodiazepines, anticholinergics. I have been very adamant about keeping Shae-Lynne away from second hand smoke. Cigarette smoke irritates the delicate lining of the esophagus making it more vulnerable to damage. It also relaxes the LES thus increasing the incidents of reflux. With the increased chance of getting asthma being so great for her I will not risk the added lung damage. Ironically, the only smoke she has ever been exposed to was when coming and going from the hospital. Since there is no smoking allowed inside the hospital everyone does it in the entryway.

Small Frequent Meals throughout the Day—Smaller and more frequent meals can reduce the pressure on the LES making reflux less likely.

Avoid Tight Clothing—For the same reasoning as above, reducing pressure on the LES.

Provide a Pacifier for Infants/Suck Hard Candy for Adults—Saliva is a natural acid neutralizer and increasing saliva production can provide relief.

Medications

If lifestyle changes alone do not work, different types of medications are prescribed to control GERD. For maximum relief, continue the lifestyle modifications while taking the medication. Remember, it's not a cure.

I know I have described Zantac, Losec and Maxeran already but for the purpose of listing treatments, please allow me to repeat myself. All of the medications listed below are adult medications.

Antacids (available in liquid or tablet form) neutralize stomach acid for up to an hour. They can interfere with the effectiveness of certain medications such as antibiotics and heart medications so always consult your doctor. They should not be given long-term or mixed with infant formula because they can result in aluminum toxicity (aluminum toxins in the system may cause adverse health conditions) and osteomalacia (soft bones). Over-the-counter antacids will help with heartburn, acid indigestion and a sour stomach.

Examples:

- Mylanta II
- Maalox
- Milk of Magnesia
- Gaviscon
- Tums
- Rolaids

H-2 blockers—(histamine receptor) block acid production in the stomach. They begin to work in about an hour and the effects can last up to twelve hours. The H-2 blockers listed below are primarily for minor symptoms caused by GER, such as heartburn and "acid stomach." It may take a few days before getting relief. H-2 blockers may not be as effective as proton pump inhibitors; however, they are very effective, safe for long-term use and less expensive. Some side effects of the H-2 receptor antagonist are headaches, dizziness, constipation, nausea/vomiting, and tiredness.

Examples:

- Pepcid (famotidine)
- Axid AC (Nizatidine): not usually for children
- Zantac (Ranitidine): most common for children
- Tagamet (Cimetidine): may cause interaction with other drugs

Proton Pump Inhibitors—Proton pump refers to the area where hydrochloric acid is produced and pumped into the stomach by these pumps. These medications almost completely shut down acid production. These drugs are prescribed when reduction of acid is required for healing. Because of the expense, H-2 blockers are usually tried before proton pump inhibitors. *Once you start a proton pump inhibitor it is usually for life.*

Examples:

- Prilosec/Losec (omeprazole)
- Nexium (made by the makers of Prilosec)
- Prevacid (Lansoprazole)
- Rabeprazole (Aciphex)
- Pantoprazole (Protonix)

Specifically, Prilosec was first introduced in 1990. Being a delayed-release tablet it will begin working within one hour, providing relief for over twenty-four hours. Unfortunately, it must be taken long term to keep the problem under control. Prilosec and Prevacid are the two commonly used in infants and children, although doctors are now beginning to use Nexium in some kids. Currently Shae-Lynne is on an adult dosage of Prilosec (Losec).

Motility Medications (Prokinetics)—These medications speed up stomach emptying time, and increase the strength of the lower esophageal sphincter (LES). If the stomach empties quickly, there is less chance of reflux. They increase the muscle tone of the digestive tract and keep the food moving better. They are also called kinetic or prokinetic agents and are usually used in combination with an H-2 blocker or proton pump inhibitor. The side affects appear to be minimal, maybe some diarrhea.

Examples:

- Reglan or Maxeran (metoclopramide)
- Ethanechol (Urecholine)
- Motilium (Domperidone)
- Propulsid (cisapride)
- Erythromycin

Reglan (metoclopramide) causes the stomach to empty quickly, thus stimulating stomach contractions. Reglan will block nausea "triggers" in the brain. A child's dose must not exceed 0.5 mg/kg, as higher doses produce symptoms similar to Parkinson's disease (tremors). Possible side effects can include depression, and potentially harmful neuromuscular problems.

Bethanochol (Urecholine) Acts on the Esophagus.

Motilium (Domperidone) acts on esophagus and stomach. Similar to Reglan wherein it helps empty the stomach more quickly; unlike Reglan it will not cross the blood-brain barrier. The side effects appear to be minimal, maybe some diarrhea. This drug is not widely used for children. This drug is not currently available in the United States.

Erythromycin is an antibiotic that in small doses has been found to promote motility.

Propulsid (cisapride) is currently off the market although it is still prescribed in some cases. Ask your doctor. It causes the LES (lower part of the esophagus) to contract. This can reduce the amount of acid that may enter the esophagus from the stomach. Caution is recommended if you do decide to try Propulsid, as it has been associated in rare cases to show abnormal heart rhythms.

Sometimes one drug may increase or decrease the effect of another drug. If your child is taking other medications, it is extremely important to check with your pharmacist for the complete listing of any drugs that may interact with the newly prescribed drug. Be sure your doctor is also aware if your child is currently taking another medication. This will ensure that the proper drug and dose will be prescribed. You should never alter the dose as prescribed by your doctor. Any signs of side affects should be carefully weighed with the benefits received. My advice is to stay well informed and you will be able to speak intelligently with your doctor. You will be able to ask the right questions and get the right answers. You need to play a major role in this. I am reminded of an exceptional doctor, Dr. Bernie Siegel (remember he sent the massage kit for Shae-Lynne) writing about "exceptional" patients. According to Dr. Siegel, these patients get involved in their own treatment. They voice their opinion. We must also stay involved and speak for our infants.

The majority of people will find sufficient relief with any one of the above-mentioned treatments.

Okay, so what happens if you are in the minority and nothing has helped you? The final option is surgery. What I have found very frustrating is that a lot of articles lack information at this point. Most simply say, "A small number may require surgery." That's it.

Well not me, here is information on the surgery, including possible complications.

Surgery or Not?

Because it is so difficult to find information on the surgery I referred back to the moms I had become friends with for the majority of my information. Their children had gone through this surgery; they gave me the pros and cons and even provided me with articles detailing it further. I learned the most common, so-called anti-reflux surgery is called a fundoplication. The Nissen version of the fundoplication has been performed since the 1950s or 60s. More is known about its effectiveness than about newer techniques. The Nissen wrap involves bringing the upper portion of the stomach (fundus) full circle around the esophagus (360) from the back (posterior) and stitching it in the front. Depending on the surgeon's preference or the patient's particular condition, there are variations to this procedure. Mainly in infants and children, a gastronomy (feeding tube or button inserted into the stomach) is usually performed at the time of a fundoplication for the purpose of feeding and venting gas.

There are complications related to the fundo. Although the majority may be performed without problems, there are children who still have symptoms or a whole new set of problems due to the surgery. From all the information I have read I have not been willing to take a chance. Luckily the doctors have recommended against it in our case.

Having said that, it is important to stress that the majority of children have no problems post fundo. This can be a life-saving surgery for many children with frequent apneas or aspiration pneumonias.

Some of drawbacks to surgery include:

Delayed Gastric Emptying (DGE)—The stomach may be slower than before to send food to the intestines or a delay that was not a big issue before can become a real problem. Pyloroplasty (stretching of the sphincter at the bottom of the stomach leading into the intestines) promotes faster emptying. However, this can cause *Dumping syndrome*, which is rapid emptying of the stomach that may cause severe nausea, abdominal cramping, retching, pale skin and sweating. Diet changes may help.

Disruption of Fundoplication—The stitches may come undone and the stomach then returns to its previous position. This will obviously leave the child back to where he/she started. One good retch has been reported to disrupt the wrap, although most reports indicate a fall or other accident may have the same affect.

Dysphagia—Swallowing is affected, along with decreased esophageal motility. Great care is taken when working near the nerves that control swallowing. Low motility and a new wrap means food gets stuck in the esophagus.

Failure to Eat Solid Meals—Certain foods may not be tolerated after surgery and therefore liquids and foods are introduced slowly. Usually a gastronomy is performed at the time of the fundo. If not, a naso-gastric tube may be placed or second surgery to insert a G-tube may be needed if the child doesn't eat properly. Fear of choking, difficulty swallowing and existing pain may cause the child to refuse food.

Gas Bloat—The inability to burp means gas must travel the length of the intestines causing pain and bloating.

Obstruction at Fundoplication—The food moves down through the esophagus but cannot pass through to the stomach.

Recurrence of Symptoms—I have found more moms than I can count whose children continue to have the same symptoms after surgery. Sometimes this is caused by a disruption of the wrap; however, many times the wrap remains intact and the children continue to experience the same problems as before the surgery.

Retching—Dry heaves.

Small Bowel Obstruction—Scar tissue can form in the abdominal cavity as a result of many surgeries. For some reason adhesions are more common after any anti-reflux procedure. If they block the passage of food through the intestines, it can require emergency surgery. The "typical" symptom of an obstruction, vomiting, may not happen after a fundoplication. Any signs of an obstruction need to be investigated immediately.

Stricture—Scarring and narrowing of esophagus. Most often this is a recurrence of scar tissue present before surgery. Even stopping acid exposure totally doesn't always prevent a recurrence.

Tube Feeding Dependence—If children are tube fed for a long period of time after surgery, it can be difficult to make the transition back to oral feeding.

Disruption of the wrap, gas bloat, obstruction, a dependence on tube feeding, strictures and the recurrence of symptoms seem to be the most common problems. These are very real possibilities. Although surgery is a final alternative when all other means have failed it is not to be taken lightly. Take the time to do your own research and draw your own conclusions to make the best decision for your child. As I said, most fundos are performed with great success but it's not likely to be a magic cure.

The following procedures are relatively new treatments for adult patients suffering from GERD. If these new procedures are as good as their claims, hopefully, they will be done in children in the near future.

Stretta—The Stretta Catheter is inserted into the patient's mouth and advanced to the junction of the esophagus and stomach (GE junction). A balloon is inflated and needle electrodes are deployed into the tissue. Radiofrequency (RF) energy is delivered through the electrodes to create thermal lesions in the muscle of the LES and gastric cardia. As these lesions heal, the tissue contracts, resulting in a reduction of reflux episodes and improvement in GERD symptoms (quoted from Curon Medical, curonmedical.com).

Endocinch—Using an endoscope the physician lowers the suturing system to the site where the esophagus and the stomach meet. The physician then places a series of two adjacent stitches below the sphincter. The two adjacent stitches below the sphincter are brought together in apposition, forming a pleat. The pleat alters the gate or valve to reduce the backflow of acid from the stomach up through the esophagus. The physician may create more than one pleat below the sphincter depending on individual circumstances (quoted from endocinch.com).

Epilogue

by Roni MacLean

When I first read *Welcome to Holland*, a poem by Emily Perl Kingsley printed at the beginning of this book, I cried. I found it very early in my research into Shae-Lynne's GERD on the personal website another mom had made for her son. He also just happened to have GERD. As I began to read, I thought how bizarre it was to have such a poem on this site; this little boy had reflux, not a disability. Yet, it so perfectly described how I had been feeling when I couldn't describe it myself. I cried because I had not yet gotten to a place where I could say I liked Holland.

When I found out I was pregnant, I was so thrilled. I didn't think anything could bring me down. A new life was beginning, a perfect new life, and the possibilities were endless. My plans were set in stone as my son/daughter was to be the smartest, cutest, healthiest, happiest baby ever. I would breast-feed for six months and that would be a breeze. I certainly read enough about it. The summer would be spent sitting by the water reading alphabet books to the baby who would surely be reading by the time he/she could talk. This is what little girls dream about from the time they are old enough to play with dolls. My biggest concern—please let her have her Auntie Michelle's beautiful curls.

When Shae-Lynne was born, life was truly bliss—for one brief moment. I looked into her tiny sweet face and felt as though I'd known her forever. At that moment I could not imagine what life was like before her. I was instantly, hopelessly and unconditionally in love.

But then something seemed amiss with our perfect plans. In the weeks and months following her birth, we seemed to be getting further and further away from our dreams. We saw doctors, nurses, nutritionists, all talking way too fast and way over our heads about things we didn't want to know about or hear. The horror of it all—hospitals, tests, medical equipment, medications and procedures were now our new life. I was crushed. Inside I was drowning in a sea of anger, resentment, guilt, exhaustion and sorrow. Outside I was trying to keep up a brave front.

I had become so focused on how things were supposed to be that I was not able to accept or even enjoy the way things were. At first, it was myself I felt sorry for and I mourned for my dream. Immediately I wanted to have another baby, another shot at getting it right. Every once in awhile I would try to imagine what it would be like if Shae-Lynne had been born healthy. Ah, life would be so easy.

After a short time of watching what Shae-Lynne was going through I started to feel sorry for her. She certainly did nothing to deserve this. It broke my heart that life for her was having a tube jammed down her throat all the time and tape across her face as it pulled and irritated her delicate skin. I hated that she had grown accustomed to the IV pole being dragged behind her everywhere she went. I dreaded that learning to walk meant learning to carry the pump and bag around with her. I knew that would also mean tripping over the tubing that inevitably dragged on the floor. It wasn't fair that her days were spent not in laughing and playing but in gagging, retching, puking and doctors. I loved Shae-Lynne more than life itself. I wanted the best for her—clearly, this was not the best life could offer.

Slowly something wonderful began to happen, just as Emily Perl Kingsley wrote. I began to look around and *Holland* really wasn't so bad. It was after all—home. Now I am able to read *Welcome to Holland* and smile.

I realized Shae-Lynne was born with a medical condition that did not make her any less perfect to me. I could not imagine loving Shae-Lynne more than I do now. It just isn't possible. I know that if she hadn't been so sick I would have gone back to work right away and missed a lot of time with her. All that we had been through made me absolutely treasure everything she accomplished. Nothing was taken for granted. Because her development was behind every new milestone was truly a Godsend. I marveled at every little thing she did with such adoration. The simplest things gave me more joy than I have ever known. Shae-Lynne has only recently started laughing and does it so seldom that it means the world to me. It can reverse even my worst mood. Her laughter is the greatest sound I hear, I still laugh out loud every time I hear it. Her speech is so incredibly far behind that I cannot even imagine what it will be like to hear her first words—a miracle.

So, I drag a feeding pump around and clean a J-tube site every day. That's life. Doesn't make it any less perfect, just different. Instead of reading alphabet books by the water, they were read in a hospital room. The scenery wasn't as nice, but at least we didn't get sunburned. Do I wish Shae-Lynne would eat? Of course, I do. Do I wish she did not feel such pain? Definitely, without a doubt! Do I walk around all day moping and feeling sorry for her? No, she doesn't need to see pity in my eyes. She needs to see love. She's not unhappy and feeling sorry for herself, so why should I? To her this is normal and she is, above all else, a happy, silly, little girl. Can I imagine her being anyone but who she is? Absolutely not! Will she ever eat? Ah, the elusive question that everyone ultimately asks. Yes, I have no doubt that she will do so someday, but until she does it is certainly not the be all and end all of my happiness. I am enjoying "the very special, the very lovely things, about *Holland.*"

Now, if I try to imagine what things would be like if Shae-Lynne had been born healthy, I cannot. Everything that has happened since her birth has made her who she is and she is my hero.

Epilogue

by Jean McNeil

Our decision to write this book was based on our desires to raise awareness, and to help those trying to cope with infant reflux not to feel so alone. We want to reach people worldwide in hopes they will share our pain and feel overwhelmed with love and want to help. Gastro Esophageal Reflux Disease *should* be a household word like cancer, diabetes, and heart attack. This disease is just as serious as the previously mentioned diseases; yet, is often dismissed as, "take an antacid" or in the case of an infant "they will outgrow it." Esophageal cancer, which is a direct result of advanced GERD, is the eighth most common cancer in the world and the sixth most common cause of death from cancer, as per the statistics from the American Cancer Society. Sounds extremely serious to me!

I think back to September 11, 2001—America's tragedy hit. Four planes were hi-jacked. Two planes were flown into the New York World Trade Center, which later crumbled to the ground. One plane hit the Pentagon in Washington, D.C., and another crashed outside of Pittsburgh, Pennsylvania. September 11, 2001, an unbelievable tragedy that is unfortunately all too real. It was clearly evident all Americans were deeply saddened by the loss, whether or not they were personally affected. Hour after hour news reporters broadcast touching stories of the victims. Family members and friends all spoke out. They shared from their hearts how much a victim had meant to them. We heard miraculous stories of survivors who somehow avoided this disastrous fate. So many people were suffering. We were all sickened. The American way of life had changed forever.

Out of this tragedy, Americans pulled together. That was what was important. Everyone joined together to help in any way they could. Millions of dollars were donated. Famous artists shared their talents to raise money. Thousands of people stood in long lines for hours to donate blood. The

President named a certain day as Prayer Day. The love shown was incredible. The terrorists hope to bring America down had the opposite effect. Everyone united.

As I lay awake and watched the sadness reported, there were tears in my eyes as one individual in particular described their pain. However, I also felt anger and thought: they are having their say. They are able to express their hurt, anger, etc. But, there is also another tragedy going on in the world every day—and it is not getting any attention.

I am talking about what this entire book is about, the infants who are suffering because of infant GERD. Their disease is not getting the attention it deserves. If you are a parent of a reflux child you know what I am saying and I am sure you feel the same frustration as I. If you have no experience with this disease, I can only pray that this book has opened your eyes and given you something to think about.

Imagine a room filled with five to six thousand infants and they all vomit and choke at the same time. They continue to choke and choke. No relief in sight. How long could you stay and watch this scene? Please picture this. It is real. It is happening all the time. Is it any less of a tragedy because it is so spread out and no one is talking about it?

I know at times I feel guilty because I am so far removed physically from Shae-Lynne and I do not have to watch her constant day-to-day suffering. I visit for a short time and hopefully Shae-Lynne isn't doing too badly that week. Just because we are not seeing something firsthand or experiencing it ourselves it *is* happening. As with America's tragedy, we all pulled together—let's join together now to help these infants.

Finally, I'd like to share with you some time I spent with Shae-Lynne. Every year I look forward to going back there, a gorgeous seaside community; after all, I lived there almost seventeen years. The beauty is just unbelievable and the quiet peaceful streets are a welcomed change to the busy city life I have been living. Now, I have all the more reason to go back. My gorgeous new granddaughter and obviously I look forward to seeing Roni and Michael, too.

As I plan my visit I see in my mind that I am arriving at the airport, Michael, Roni and Shae-Lynne are there to meet me. I picture sweet little Shae-Lynne walking toward me with a huge smile on her face and her arms extended reaching for me. I picture this over and over in my mind. I dream for this to be a reality. I so want for her to like me. Roni had told me Shae-Lynne is taking her first steps. She is still very nervous, I believe, because of the tube and pump she is hooked up to all the time. They must be a weight that makes her uncomfortable.

Shae-Lynne has been through so much. So many hospital stays. So many strangers (nurses, doctors, etc.) have hurt her in the attempts to bring her relief. I realize that I too am just another stranger to her.

I decided to arrive at the airport with what would be Shae-Lynne's first doll. If I bribed her maybe she would like me. She wanted no part of her new doll. Roni thought maybe she was jealous of it. I was just pleased that Shae-Lynne seemed happy to see me. I knew it would take a few days for her to get closer to me and that would require patience on my part. I think she knew my voice. We talked on the phone all the time. Well actually I talk and she listens and plays with the buttons on the phone.

Roni had called me many times, "Another bad morning, Mom. Shae-Lynne threw up four times already today." Each and every call I received was so hard because I was unable to help. I knew Roni was hurting and I knew Shae-Lynne hurt, too. Now that I was with them I wanted to do something to help yet I couldn't because Shae-Lynne only wanted Mommy. I knew I must give Shae-Lynne the time to get to know me, but I wanted so badly to grab her in my arms and hug her to pieces. I tried to sneak little hugs and kisses and each time Roni would run for the camera. Hopefully, one photo would turn out nice.

Shae-Lynne was still borderline failure to thrive. She was so tiny and fragile. The average baby takes a fall, gets up and keeps on going. To Shae-Lynne, a little stumble was so devastating. She would become so upset for the longest time and she only wanted Mommy. Well, sometimes Daddy would do, but mostly it was Mommy and only Mommy. Didn't leave Roni much time for herself! A few tumbles that Shae-Lynne took I couldn't help but wonder had her feeding tube pulled and irritated her site.

Roni often told me she felt guilty as she may be spoiling Shae-Lynne. I think she was only giving her love. I felt when the time was important Roni would know when to say "no" to Shae-Lynne and mean it. I think I was fooling myself, as I may have believed "she would grow out of this by now." I was thinking that once the tube was gone....

When the average baby cries or throws a tantrum because they are not getting their own way sometimes you just let them cry it out. You must to show that your "no" means "no." Another example may be when you place your infant in their crib for a nap and they do not settle. It is perfectly fine to let them fuss awhile. With Shae-Lynne, Roni could not do that. It is extremely difficult when you have an infant that must not get upset. If Shae-Lynne got the least bit upset she would choke more. What a predicament Roni had to deal with.

On my first day there, I took Shae-Lynne for a stroll around town in her carriage. As long as Shae-Lynne was in the carriage and busy, Roni could have a much-needed hour break. Off we went, walking the boardwalk together. I wanted so much to enjoy this; however, I was really nervous. I couldn't help but wonder: What if the feeding pump beeps? What if Shae-Lynne starts to vomit? What if she starts to choke? What should I do if the tube gets air in it or kinks? What if the formula gets plugged and isn't feeding through the tube properly? Wow, so much could go wrong. I am not the nervous type, not a worrier at all, and here I was feeling queasy in my stomach over what should be a pleasant stroll. It was such a gorgeous day and I was where I wanted to be, with my sweet granddaughter, alongside this breathtaking scenery. Yet, I feared what may happen. I decided it was best to stay close to their home. Roni had a nice shower, Shae-Lynne had a nice walk and I ended up with a migraine. Our next walk, I was somewhat braver and more at ease so we went further from home.

Because of lack of space, Michael graciously offered up his place in bed and settled for the sofa during my visit. Shae-Lynne had been so traumatized by the surgery done to perform the insertion of the J-tube that Michael and Roni had taken her into their bed. Now here I was beside Shae-Lynne each night. She was getting to know me. With the nightlight on and the streetlight shining in our window, I would lay and watch her fall asleep. I would finally start to relax then I'd notice Shae-Lynne open her eyes and I would feel her reach over and ever so gently touch my cheek and grab my nose and hair. I am sure she wondered who this strange lady was in Daddy's place. As she glanced over, our eyes met just as I had dreamt about. Shae-Lynne suddenly gave me that huge smile of hers. She touched my hair once again. She rolled onto her other side quickly just checking to be sure her mommy was there. I smiled and felt tears in my eyes. I loved the moonlight shining in our window. I felt overwhelmed with love.

Only seconds before the smile Shae-Lynne was vomiting and choking. I guess you can get used to seeing the constant vomiting, but the choking was another thing. She choked and strained to get the bile up. She had no food in her stomach as the feeding tube was in her bowel. It would not come. Shae-Lynne cried harder. She struggled to breathe. The vomit just would not come up. She was so uncomfortable. The tears streamed down her cheeks. Roni was holding Shae-Lynne in her arms rocking her. I was trying to hold towels to catch the vomit. Shae-Lynne continued to cry, she thrust her whole body back with such force that it was hard for Roni to hold onto her. Still trying to hold towels in place, I wound up the music box to help relax her. The choking and vomiting continued for a while. Finally we thought this episode might be over.

"Damn it, Roni, I want someone to film this. People need to see this."

Roni sadly stated, "What for, Mom? No one will look. No one cares." We sat in silence as tears rolled down our cheeks. Roni continued to rock and cuddle Shae-Lynne. We were sitting in bed at one a.m. living our own little hell. Roni was crying. She was crying from exhaustion. This was a nightly occurrence for them. She was crying for Shae-Lynne's suffering. We lay tensed as the minutes pass. We were waiting for the next vomiting attack and praying that it did not come.

Things settled down for a while. Roni and I both lay awake watching beautiful innocent Shae-Lynne. Why does she have to suffer so? As Shae-Lynne began to dose off, beep, beep, beep goes her pump. The tube got kinked. Roni gently raises Shae-Lynne higher onto the pillow, as an infant with reflux must stay elevated so that her lungs will stay clear. It seemed as through things may be okay now. It was approaching two a.m. and Roni had to get up and add formula to Shae-Lynne's feeding bag.

The formula could only be at room temperature for approximately four hours. Beep, beep, beep—yes, it was time for more formula. Very quietly Roni sneaked downstairs hoping not to disturb Shae-Lynne.

Coming onto a new day, the sun had risen and it was gorgeous outside. I could see the lake and all the boats. I whispered loving thoughts to Shae-Lynne, thinking surely this would be a better day.

It saddened me so to know that Roni, Michael and Shae-Lynne go through this so often. I cannot imagine what it must be like for both Roni and Michael to watch their beautiful new child suffer and not be able to help. I feel guilty, as I would leave in a few days. As the saying goes: *out of sight, out of mind.* Would this horrible night leave me? I don't think so. However, I would not have to watch it nightly, or every morning as they do.

Unfortunately, morning was always the worst, I assume because Shae-

Lynne had been fairly still all night. The choking would start all over again. All we can do is "wait for her to outgrow this." I try to believe this "will outgrow" thing and yet I remember reading, "once a patient is prescribed this medication…—*it is for life!*"

FREQUENTLY ASKED QUESTIONS

At what age does reflux tend to peak? When will it get better?

Generally, it is said that in normal cases of reflux it will peak between four and six months. These normal cases of reflux tend to improve around seven to nine months and completely outgrow it by one year. Cases like Shae's that are much more serious and classified as GERD may last until eighteen months or two years. If reflux lasts beyond two years it is likely that it will continue through childhood.

Should I breast-feed my refluxer? Does breast-feeding make it worse?

Breast-feeding is highly beneficial for reflux and GERD. Whey, the protein in breast milk, is much easier to digest than casein, the protein found in formula. It empties from the stomach up to twice as fast as formula, and that can help prevent reflux and the accompanying acid pain and vomiting. Breast-fed babies tend to eat smaller meals more frequently than their formula-fed peers, which can also help decrease reflux episodes.

Breast-feeding also helps prevent food allergies. Breast milk helps to protect the intestines, coating them with an immunoglobulin called secretory IGA and keeping allergens out of the bloodstream.

My baby seemed to be improving and now we are going downhill again, what caused this?

As stated above, reflux tends to peak between four and six months, this could be why you are seeing an increase in reflux activity. Perhaps you have introduced a new food that is not agreeing with your child. Think about what he/she has eaten in the last twenty-four hours. Have they gained weight? Perhaps an increase in medication would be beneficial. Stomach bugs, colds, teething, anything like that can make reflux worse. The most important thing to remember is that reflux does, for whatever reason, tend to leave your child on a roller coaster of good days/weeks and bad days/weeks. Try to think about some of the things I mentioned but don't drive yourself nuts trying to figure out why, because you probably never will.

Prevacid/Prilosec, which is better?

Really neither, everyone is different. Some parents will swear by Prilosec, some will swear by Prevacid.

My baby was a good eater but recently has started refusing food and taking less and less. What should I do?

Keep a dairy of intake and watch your baby's weight. Do everything you can in terms of medication to control the pain from reflux and that should be enough to get your baby eating again. If it is not, continue with a detailed diary of eating patterns. Get a consult with a pediatric dietician or nutritionist to get an idea what he should be eating and compare that with your diary. Above all, in my opinion, do not force feed. This can cause oral aversions and increase their anxiety around eating, that's the last thing you need.

My baby was put on Zantac; will this help with the throwing up?

Probably not. It's an acid reducer only, which means it should help with the possible pain from acid burning but won't make the refluxing or throwing up stop.

My baby cries all the time. How do I know if it's reflux or colic?

Personally, I believe that many so-called colicky babies are really undiagnosed refluxers. Watch for other symptoms of reflux like throwing up, fussiness after eating, back arching, sour breath, congestion, apnea, and frequent chest infections. If your baby seems more comfortable sleeping upright, being carried, or lying on the stomach it could be reflux. Does he/she seem to eat small, but frequent meals? Try some lifestyle adjustments: (1) keep him/her upright for at least thirty minutes after a feeding, (2) keep baby in a bouncy chair or swing which allows him to be upright but doesn't put too much pressure on his belly, (3) avoid clothes that are constrictive in the belly, and (4) try adjusting his sleeping positions by keeping him propped up. Discuss sleeping positions with your doctor; many times refluxers prefer sleeping on their belly. (Important: Do not put your baby on its belly without consulting your ped first, it can put them at an increased risk for SIDS). Trust your instincts, if you believe that your baby has reflux consult your pediatrician armed with your list of symptoms.

Is reflux genetic?

Yes. PAGER (Pediatric and Adolescent Gastro Esophageal Reflux Association) has funded a research program that suggests a gene for severe pediatric GER maps to chromosome 13q14.

My baby is on a proton pump inhibitor but is still miserable. How do I know if it's working?

Generally, if you have given the proton pump inhibitor for at least a week (or whatever your doctor suggests) and have not seen results it's a good guess that it's not working. Consult your pediatrician; he may try a different proton pump inhibitor. A pH-probe (test where a tube is inserted into the esophagus to measure the amount of acid that makes contact with it in a 24-hour period of time) is an option. I used litmus paper with Shae a couple times. If I happen to see a good sample of clear vomit come up I will stick a little piece of litmus paper (found at the local drug store) in the vomit to see if it's acidic. I don't know how accurate this method is. I've never heard of anyone else trying it; however, I do know that when she was screaming and writhing in pain I got an acidic result (under four) and when she was going through a good spell of not exhibiting pain it came up neutral (four and above). If you decide to try this at home make sure to test only clear fluid or the color of the liquid may interfere with your results.

My baby screams all day but is gaining weight so my ped won't listen to me. What should I do to help him/her?

Try all the lifestyle changes listed and everything that you can do yourself without the doctor's advice first. If none of that helps, try videotaping your baby and take that to the child's doctor. Perhaps that will make him listen. If all your attempts to get through to your doctor fail, maybe you should consider another doctor's opinion.

I can't stand this, I am so sick of cleaning puke. What can I do?

If you've done everything you can by way of treatments and lifestyle changes, basically the answer is there is nothing you can do but continue to clean puke and wait. Just remember that as bad as you feel right now, and as hard as it is to get through one more episode of screaming, or throwing up, you will get through it. You will get through it because you have to. Get online, if possible, for emotional support.

What is the best formula to feed my reflux baby?

Breast milk. Besides that, there really isn't one formula that is better than another. This, as with the medication, is purely going to depend on your child, because everyone is different. Often reflux is caused or made worse by milk allergies, and any of the following hypo-allergenic formulas may help: Nutramigen, Alimentum, Pregestimil, Neocate, and Vivonex. These are not always necessary; some kids improve by simply switching to soy-based formulas. Enfamil came out with a formula specifically to help with throwing up, in which they added rice starch, called Enfamil AR. If you see that one is not working, consult your ped about trying another. They generally say to give it a week or so to be able to tell if your child will tolerate a new formula. With Shae, we knew within 20 minutes if the change in formula was going to work or not. Trust your instincts; the doctor has the degree, but you have the child every day, all day.

My baby seems to be throwing up more now after just having had a G-tube operation. Is this normal?

Yes. Gastronomies can definitely make reflux worse and in some cases even cause reflux when there was previously no history of the problem. This surgery increases the pressure inside the stomach and on the LES making reflux episodes more common. Most surgeons will not even perform a gastronomy without also performing a fundo at the same time, even if there is no history of reflux, just as a preventative measure.

Best wishes to you all!

GLOSSARY

Acid reflux—Muscular valve (L.E.S.) at the end of esophagus relaxes to often, allowing the stomach acid to escape.

ALTE—Apparent life-threatening events

Amino acids—Basic building blocks of proteins. The body makes many amino acids, others come from food and the body breaks them down for use by cells.

Aspirate—Food or refluxed material goes into the lungs

Barrett's Esophagus—Constant irritation from stomach acid causes this serious condition. The tissues lining the esophagus become abnormal, which may eventually develop into esophageal cancer.

Biopsies—removal of a small piece of living tissue from the body for examination under a microscope

Celiac Disease—sensitivity of the small intestines to gluten, a protein found in rye, wheat and barley. The sensitivity causes an inability to absorb nutrients due to inflammation and damage to the intestinal lining.

D.G.E.—Delayed gastric emptying. The food does not empty into the intestines as fast as it should, thus leaving the child feeling full longer.

Duodenum—Uppermost part of small intestines

Dysphagia—difficulty swallowing

Esophagus—Long muscular tube connecting the mouth and stomach

Esophagitis—Inflammation and damage to the lining of the esophagus

Failure to Thrive—FTT occurs when an infant, toddler, or child fails to grow at a normal rate. This may be due to environmental causes or genetics. FTT is diagnosed when the child's weight is below the 5th percentile.

Fluoroscopy—a diagnostic procedure in which x-rays that have passed through the body are projected onto a screen, providing continuous image of the body's internal structures

Fundoplication—so-called anti-reflux surgery

Fundus—upper portion of the stomach

Gastroenterologist—a physician who specializes in disorders of the gastro intestinal tract, including stomach, intestines, and associated organs

Gastronomy—surgically produced opening in stomach, usually connects the stomach to the outside so that a feeding tube can be placed in the stomach or passed into the small intestine. The process of inserting a G-tube.

Geneticist—one who studies genetics/heredity

Heartburn—Burning pain caused by acid from the stomach flowing into the esophagus. It is a symptom of reflux.

Hydrochloric Acid—Acid produced by the stomach to digest food

Jejunostomy—Surgery to insert a tube into the side of the belly directly into the jejunum. The process of inserting a J-tube.

Laparoscopic—Describes a way to perform surgery in which small punctures are made in the abdomen permitting insertion of a telescope for viewing and instruments to do an operation

L.E.S.—lower esophageal sphincter valve; when working properly, allows food, water, etc. to pass into the stomach; and prevents backward flow of stomach acid

N G Tube—Used as a means of feeding. N—naso, meaning through the nose and G—gastric, meaning into the stomach.

N J Tube—Used as a means of feeding. N—naso, meaning through the nose and J—down into the jejunum (second part of the small bowel)

Neonatologist—branch of pediatrics—concerned with care of newborn infants and treatment of their disorders

Nutritionist—specialized science and study of foodstuff people eat and drink and the way they are digested and assimilated

Pyloric Stenosis—Muscle at the bottom of the stomach is too thick or blocked

Silent Reflux—reflux that occurs without symptoms, i.e., vomiting, etc.

Stricture—A narrowing of a hollow organ of the body, such as the esophagus

TESTS

Barium Swallow—(see upper G.I.)

Blood Count—measures hemoglobin concentration, and number of red blood cells, white cells and platelets in one cubic millimeter of blood

E.E.G.—Electroencephalogram, a type of brainwave analysis that shows certain characteristic patterns if an individual has seizures or some abnormality in the brain

E.K.G.—Electrocardiogram, electric recording of the heart

Electrolytes—Chemicals such as salts and minerals needed for various functions in the body.

Endoscopy—Reveals extent of damage done by reflux. A flexible tube (endoscope) with lights and a camera is passed down the child's mouth into the esophagus, stomach, and duodenum. The doctor can look directly at the esophagus, stomach and duodenum to see if any damage is present. The doctor can also take a biopsy at this time.

M.R.I.—Magnetic Resonance Imaging. MRI is a diagnostic technique that provides high quality cross-sectional images of organs and structures within the body and without x-ray or other radiation

R.A.S.T. (allergy)—Radioallergosorbent test—a blood test. If positive, it indicates that a person is allergic to the particular substance tested, such as a specific food, mold, dust or pollen

Reflux Scan—Similar to upper G.I. Child swallows barium, is laid flat on a table which has an x-ray under it. The x-ray takes constant pictures for one hour to measure amount of reflux.

Upper G.I. (barium swallow)—Child swallows a small amount of radioactive solution called barium, the doctor watches a series of fluoroscopy x-rays. The barium highlights or outlines the esophagus, throat and upper intestines which allows the doctor to view the food as it travels down the esophagus into the stomach and into the first part of the small intestines.

Ultrasound—Procedure combines high frequency sound waves and computer technology to provide pictures of your internal organs.

DRUGS

Antacid—Reduces stomach acid

Acid Blocker—A drug prescribed to suppress the amount of acid in the stomach so that what is being refluxed and or vomited is not so acidic and would not irritate or inflame the esophagus

Histamine H-2 Receptor; Receptor/Antagonist or Blocker—Medications that prevents stimulation of the acid producing cells in the stomach

Losec (Omeprazole) (Canadian) and Prilosec (US)—See Proton pump inhibitor

Maxeran (Reglan) (Metoclopramide)—See Prokinetic

Motilium—Acts on esophagus and stomach—similar to Prokinetic, helps empty stomach more quickly.

Prokinetic—Increases gastric emptying time. Causing the stomach to empty faster and increases the strength of the LES

Proplusid (Cisapride)—See Prokinetic

Proton Pump Inhibitor—Proton pump refers to the site in stomach cell where hydrochloric acid is produced and pumped into stomach. (Inhibitor—meaning slowing or preventing the production of acid in the stomach.) Example: Losec

Zantac (Ranitidine)—Is an acid blocker or Histamine H-2 receptor

SUGGESTED READING

Coping with Chronic Heartburn—What You Need to Know About Acid Reflux and GERD
Elaine Fantle Shimberg
St Martins Griffin 2001

Freedom from Digestive Distress—Medicine-Free Relief
Gary Gitnick, MD with Karen Cooksey
The Three Rivers Press TM of Random House 2000

Is This Your Child? Discovering and Treating Unrecognized Allergies
Doris Rapp, MD
William Morrow and Company, Inc., NY 1991

Mayo Clinic on Digestive Health
John E King, MD, Editor-in-Chief
Kensington Publishing, NY 2000

Preemies—The Essential Guide for Parents of Premature Babies
Dana Wechsler Linden, Emma Trenti Paroli, Mia Wechsler Doron, MD
PocketBooks, a division of Simon & Schuster, Inc. 2000

The Fire Inside—Extinguishing Heartburn and Related Symptoms
M. Michael Wolfe, MD, and Thomas J. Nessi
W.W. Norton & Company, New York, London 1996

Signing for Kids (a fun way to learn American Sign Language)
Mickey Flodin
The Berkley Publishing Company 1991

The Out-of-Sync Child—Recognizing and Coping with Sensory Integration Dysfunction
Carol Stock Kranowitz, M.A.
The Berkley Publishing Group, 1998

You Will Dream New Dreams—Inspiring Personal Stories by Parents of Children With Disabilities
Stanley D Klein, Ph.D. and Kim Schive
Kensington Books, NY, 2001

INFORMATION AND SUPPORT

www.infantrefluxdisease.com
Shae-Lynne's personal website

Acurian, Inc
2 Walnut Grove Dr., Ste 375
Horsham, PA 19044
215-323-9125
www.acurian.com

www.g-tube.com
Denise Boyd
1802 Phillips Springs Road
Gladewater, TX 75647
Ph: 903-844-8272

IFFGD
International Foundation for Functional
Gastrointestinal Disorders, Inc.
P O Box 170864
Milwaukee, WI 53217-8076
888-964-2001
or
158 Pleasant Street
North Andover, MA 01845
800-394-2747
www.iffgd.org

Kids with Tubes
info@kidswithtubes.org

La Leche League International
1400 N Meacham Road
Schaumburg, IL 60168-4079
847-519-7730
www.lalecheleague.org

National Digestive Disease Information Clearinghouse
2 Information Way
Bethesda, MD 20892-3570
800-891-5389 or 301-654-3810

National Institute of Diabetes and Digestive and Kidney Disease
NIDDK, NIH
31 Center Drive,
Bethesda, MD 20892-2560
301-496-3583
nddic@info.niddk.nih.gov

New Visions
1124 Roberts Mountain Road
Faber, VA 22938
434-361-2285
Catalogue available

Pediatric/Adolescent Gastroesophageal
Reflux Association, Inc. (PAGER)
P O Box 1153
Germantown, MD 20875-1153
301-601-9541 or 760-747-5001
www.reflux.org
Sensory Integration International—The Ayres Clinic
1514 Cabrillo Avenue
Torrance, CA 90501
301-787-8805

The American College of Gastroenterology
4900-B South 31st Street
Arlington, VA 22206-1656
703-820-7400
800-478-2876 (information line)
www.acg.gi.org

HELPFUL CATALOGUES

Super Duper Publications
Fun Education Materials
800-277-8737
Dept SD 2002
P O Box 24997
Greenville, SC 29616-2497

Sammons Preston
P O Box 5071
Bolingbrook, IL 60440-5071
800-323-5547 or 800-325-1745
www.sammonspreston.com

CANADIAN SITES

CDDF National Office
The Canadian Digestive Disease Foundation
2702 South Sheridan Way
Oakville, Ontario
L6J 7L6
866-819-2333
E-mail: CDDFoffice@CDDF.ca

The Northwestern Society of Intestinal Research
855 West 12th Avenue
Vancouver, British Columbia
V5Z 1M9
604-875-4875
E-mail: nsir@badgut.com

Printed in the United Kingdom
by Lightning Source UK Ltd.
104928UKS00001B/313